Your Pregnancy

Month by Month

Your Pregnancy

Month by Month

Fifth Edition

Clark Gillespie, M.D.

HarperPerennial
A Division of HarperCollinsPublishers

HarperCollins books may be purchased for educational, business, or sales promotional use. For information please write: Special Markets Department, HarperCollins Publishers, Inc., 10 East 53rd Street, New York, NY 10022.

FIRST EDITION

Designed by Jessica Shatan

Library of Congress Cataloging-in-Publication Data

Gillespie, Clark
    Your pregnancy month by month / Clark Gillespie. —5th ed.
        p.   cm.
    Includes index.
    ISBN 0-06-095714-X
    1. Pregnancy—Popular works. 2. Obstetrics—Popular works
I. Title
RG525.G513 1998
618.2'4—dc21   98-18284

98 99 00 01 02 ❖/RRD 10 9 8 7 6 5 4 3

This Book Is Dedicated to
My Beloved Wife, Susan

Contents

Acknowledgments

The author is indebted to many people for assistance during this revision. In particular:

Berton Whitaker, Director, Southeast Georgia Regional Medical Center, Brunswick, Georgia.

D. Hubert Manning, M.D., Chief, Department of Radiology, and Kevin Harlan and his staff of ultrasonographers at the Southeast Georgia Regional Medical Center.

Carl W. Dohn, Jr., M.D., and his ultrasonographer, Julie Moseley.

Marijo Norris and Radiology Associates, Little Rock, Arkansas.

Steven R. Goldstein, M.D., and Contemporary OB/GYN.

Meagan Prest and the Acuson Corporation.

Andy Levy and the Corometrics Medical Systems.

Megan Newman, editor, and Hillary Epstein, editorial assistant—my guardians at HarperCollins.

Introduction to the Fifth Edition

Pregnancy is a fundamental physiological cascade that flows very powerfully in the mainstream of our lives. This vital rite of passage, so to speak, has existed as long as we have—and just as that pregnancy cascade has always been, it so remains. What, then, could require, over a few short decades, five revisions of a self-help pregnancy book such as ours?

PLENTY!

Conception, pregnancy, labor, and delivery proceed, as we have just said, in the same order and structure that they have followed since Adam and Eve. These central events are not likely to change—ever. But pregnancy, as nature designed it, can be a harsh physiological event. We have only to look back a few short intervals of time to bear out that fact. Maternal and fetal mortality in the early part of our century would blanch the most callous observer today. Just consider that as recently as fifty years ago, one mother in every ten expired during or after a cesarean section—an operation then, as now, designed to protect women in abnormal labor. Newborn infants fared even worse. But, thanks to many resources, those days are safely behind us.

Even so, there is still much to do. As physicians, our major goal has always been to make childbearing as safe as humanly possible. To this end, new procedures are constantly being introduced and confirmed or rejected. These fresh procedures must be explained in our updated book. Likewise, new risks are constantly surfacing to challenge our goals. These, too, must be faced, dealt with, and explained to you in reasonable and clear terms. That's what the fifth edition is all about.

I will try to explain these procedures and processes that affect the course of pregnancy in an enjoyable and understandable format. This book should carry readers securely into the next millennium. Let's see how we make out together.

TELEPHONE LIST

Doctor's office_____

_____

Home_____

_____

Answering service_____

_____

Hospital_____

_____

Pharmacy_____

_____

My mother_____

_____

His mother_____

_____

_____

_____

Ambulance_____

_____

Taxi_____

_____

One

My First Lunar Month

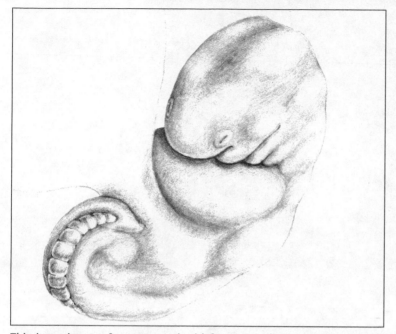

This is a picture of a one-month-old fetus. It is far from being formed and still shows evidence of rudimentary gills and a tail. The heart is beating (and can often be seen under very high resolution ultrasound) and brain centers are well established. Rudimentary eye spots can be seen. Less than half an inch long, the fetus is still attached to a yolk sac that provides very concentrated nourishment. It is hard to believe at this point that we are looking at what will be, at the end of ten lunar months, a fully formed beautiful baby! But—we are.

The accompanying ultrasound picture taken at this time reveals a dark, round yolk sac with a small signet (arrow), comprising the above-pictured little human structure.

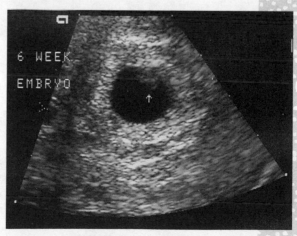

t's a done deal! A baby is on the way.

Although you did not realize it, day 1 (or night 1)—the first 24 hours of your pregnancy and your baby's existence—have just gone by. Sometime during those hours, conception occurred.

Your pregnancy began at the time of ovulation, about two weeks after the first day of your preceding menstrual period. Let's see how the whole miracle gets going.

Implantation of a Pregnancy

Each month an egg is released from one ovary or the other by the process of ovulation, and it migrates into one of the two narrow fallopian tubes that lead to the uterus. There, if the egg comes in contact with sperm that have migrated up from the vagina, fertilization occurs. After fertilization, the beginning embryo continues down into the uterus, or womb, where several days later it slips into a lush, sugar-rich bed and there grows for some 265 days. The womb's inviting lining, having received and engulfed the embryo, remains intact in order to nourish it. Thus, menstruation—the monthly shedding of this lining when it is not needed for a fertilized egg—does not occur. So the first and most common sign of pregnancy is the absence of menstruation.

Early Pregnancy Impact

The established pregnancy, new and infinitely small though it is, soon leads to awesome changes within you. These changes are instituted by certain cells that constitute part of the new life within you. These cells, called chorionic villi, are responsible, as we shall soon see, for a positive pregnancy test. Chorionic cells stimulate intense activity in the master pituitary gland and it, in turn, sends signals of impending changes to all parts of the body, as a national tracking system might alert everyone that an alien—but friendly—spaceship has landed.

One major pituitary signal alerts the corpus luteum cyst on your ovary to keep on going. This cyst forms regularly each month at the point on the ovary where ovulation took place. Usually it survives about two weeks, and its demise signals the onset of menstruation. When you are pregnant, however, your pituitary alerts the corpus luteum to stay on working in the ovary. Thus, in pregnancy this normal cyst lasts for about three months, making large amounts of the hormone progesterone. Progesterone is a fundamental hormone throughout most of your life, but at this time it prevents your uterus from rejecting your infant—which is akin to a foreign graft on your body. We want to remember that fact because it has some important implications later on. Soon the infant's placenta takes over the progesterone task, and so, by the third month, the corpus luteum withers away.

Although this cyst is a normal and absolutely necessary ovarian substance, it can cause some discomfort for you during its three-month duration—particularly some pain on the side where it develops. This pain can sometimes be confused with that of an ectopic pregnancy—a disorder explained later in this chapter.

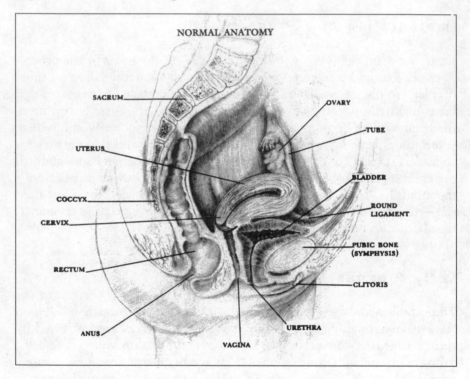

NORMAL ANATOMY

SACRUM

OVARY

TUBE

UTERUS

BLADDER

COCCYX

ROUND LIGAMENT

CERVIX

PUBIC BONE (SYMPHYSIS)

RECTUM

CLITORIS

ANUS

URETHRA

VAGINA

Signs and Symptoms of Pregnancy

The following symptoms are common signs of pregnancy:

- •**Missed period.** Many things interfere with normal menses, such as stress, exercise, illness, and so on, but a missed period is commonly the first indication of a pregnancy.

- **Engorged and tender breasts.** Breast discomfort at this time is generally greater than is usually felt just before a normal period.

- **Digestive problems.** Nausea and even vomiting are not uncommon. A smoke-filled room, which you should avoid anyway, will make you gag. Even foods you usually like may repel your sensitive stomach.

- **Fatigue.** You may find yourself becoming exhausted more easily and more frequently.

- **Repeated need to urinate.** Because of local congestion, your bladder feels full and you will urinate much more often during the day and, unfortunately, during the night as well.

- **Emotions.** You may experience moments of inexplicable depression and irritability.

Pregnancy Testing

From the dawn of time—or at least since humans became involved in it— the early determination of the existence of a pregnancy, which has such enormous social, physiological, and emotional impact, has generated fantastic interest. In ancient cultures, all manner of tests were devised to determine pregnancy. The saliva from a pregnant woman would supposedly make a goat throw up. A golden ring suspended over a woman's abdomen would spin wildly if she was pregnant—in one direction if it was a boy, another if it was a girl. One hundred and fifty years ago, the first urine pregnancy test was devised. After the urine lay flat on a plate for a few hours, it became covered with a misty, iridescent film, which sank to the bottom in five more days!

Modern medicine's romance with pregnancy testing began when it was determined that a substance secreted by the human embryo called human chorionic gonadotropin (HCG) begins to circulate in maternal blood very early on. It was also established that HCG was concentrated and excreted in maternal urine. This very specific hormone substance is secreted by embryonic chorionic villi cells almost from the moment of conception, and its secretion increases, doubling just about every other day, reaching a peak at somewhere between days 60 and 80 of pregnancy, falling rapidly thereafter, but continuing to be secreted until delivery and for several weeks following.

Since HCG is concentrated in maternal urine, early pregnancy testing was carried out on concentrated urine samples. In fact, most office tests and all home pregnancy tests still are based on that principle. In the beginning, maternal urine was injected into rabbits and, later on, into frogs in order for HCG to stimulate activity in these animals' reproductive glands.

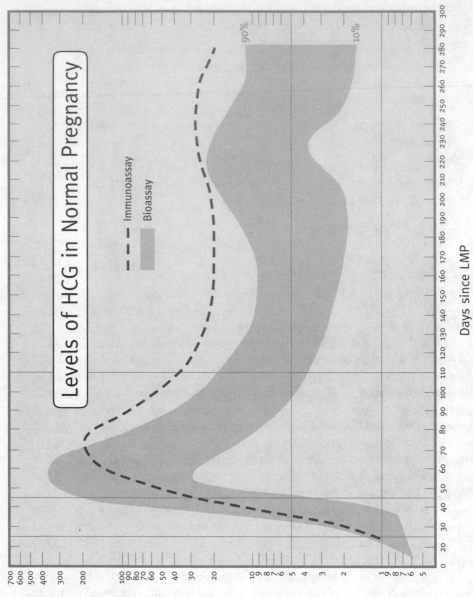

Levels of HCG in Normal Pregnancy

- - - Immunoassay
▨ Bioassay

90%

10%

Days since LMP

HCG in Thousands of IU

HCG levels (including beta HCG) rise very regularly and sharply in the normal early pregnancy days, making such levels excellent evidence of pregnancy health. Bioassay and immunoassay are just different measuring techniques. Urine testing is an example of immunoassay testing. HCG is detectable throughout pregnancy and for several weeks after delivery.

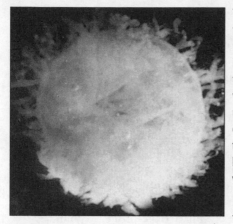

This is a total pregnancy of 26 days duration. The embryo is enclosed by a surrounding membranous chorionic sac, which
itself is seen completely coated by a multitude of hairy projections—the chorionic
villi. Some of these villi will attach to the
mother's uterine lining and form the placenta. The unattached villi areas will eventually wither away. Until they do, they can
be sampled for genetic studies—chorionic
villi sampling (CVS; see pages 283–284).
(Courtesy of Contemporary OB/GYN *and*
Steven R. Goldstein, M.D.)

Such tests were time-consuming, expensive, not uniformly accurate, and
destructive to rabbits and frogs! Today's chemical tests on urine are considerably more accurate, particularly if the urine is concentrated. The tests
are based on a complement fixation procedure—a rather complex interaction. The test is prepared as follows: In the laboratory, red blood cells are
coated with the antigen HCG. These cells clump together when and if the
antibody to HCG is added to them, unless that antibody is quickly inactivated by some other HCG antigen. Home pregnancy kits contain the
coated red blood cells and the antibody—both waiting side by side to be
moistened and mixed by urine. That is where pregnant urine comes in: it
contains the HCG antigen. Thus, home pregnancy test devices, when
moistened thoroughly with urine from a pregnant woman, do not allow
the red blood cells to clump because the urine neutralizes the test's HCG
antibody. If clumping does occur, the test is negative: either pregnancy
does not exist or the urine specimen does not contain enough HCG antigen to neutralize. (In other words, it is too early in the pregnancy or the
urine is too diluted.) The clumping—or lack of it—is made to appear in
the test window as a color or a stripe of some sort. Got all that?

Done according to the accompanying instructions, home pregnancy
tests are very accurate, very early in pregnancy.

Blood pregnancy tests, on the other hand, involve a radioimmunoassay
process that measures very accurately the presence of HCG in maternal
blood serum. Such tests are often positive within a few days after conception, but their accuracy may not be reliable until shortly after the first
missed period.

Beta HCG

The beta HCG substance provides the most valuable diagnostic pregnancy
test available today. Beta HCG, one tiny spectrum of the whole HCG

complex, is very specific for pregnancy. If there are more than three units of beta HCG in the maternal serum, pregnancy exists or has very recently existed. Our knowledge of beta HCG can help us do the following:

•Establish a very early, reliable diagnosis of pregnancy.

•Determine pregnancy health. As we have already noted, the beta subunit fraction should double almost every other day for the first 60–80 days, and as long as this is so, the pregnancy is generally healthy (see page 6). If beta HCG stops doubling with reasonable regularity, we suspect that something may have happened to the fetus within the uterus, or, of equal importance, that the pregnancy may be abnormally located somewhere outside the uterus. Therefore, the test is of real value in following high-risk, miscarriage-prone pregnancies and also in helping to determine the presence of an ectopic pregnancy and the activity within that pregnancy.

•Diagnose a very rare condition, called a hydatid mole, in which the placental cells have become highly abnormal. Such a mole may even go on to form a very rare, once deadly cancer known as chorio-carcinoma. This pregnancy test can follow the course of such extremely unusual placental abnormalities, which, fortunately, respond almost without fail to modern chemotherapy.

A variety of pregnancy tests are available for use in your home, your doctor's office, or a hospital laboratory. There are also a number of social and medical reasons for learning, at an early date, whether a pregnancy exists. Let's look at some examples:

•The absolute diagnosis of pregnancy is particularly important for someone with irregular menstrual periods who is having some symptoms of trouble such as spotting and/or pain, or if it is suspected that a pregnancy may exist outside the uterus.

•Early diagnosis is important in high-risk pregnancies. The very sensitive beta HCG test is used to follow the pregnancies of women with a history of repeated miscarriages, and pregnancies where there is a problem with spotting or pain, in order to determine for certain whether fetal life persists. The beta HCG test is also used, as we shall see, to follow the outcome of ectopic pregnancies.

•It is essential to have a test result as early as possible if an abortion is being contemplated. The sooner the diagnosis is made, the simpler and safer the procedure.

•It is important to have the diagnosis confirmed if distant or prolonged travel is anticipated so that proper precautions can be taken.

•Since certain drugs and certain X-ray examinations can interfere
with or damage a pregnancy in the early stages, pregnancy should
be confirmed. Elective surgery should also be avoided.

•The diagnosis is important where there are rubella (German
measles) epidemics. Rubella is dangerous to the fetus. Women who
might be pregnant and who have no immunity to the disease
should have the diagnosis confirmed so they can get away from
that environment as soon as possible.

•An early diagnosis can lead to an early start in appropriate prenatal
care.

How Reliable Are Home Pregnancy Tests?

About one-third of those women who think they may be pregnant try a
home pregnancy test. Manufacturers claim that such tests are at least 97
percent accurate. That is true—in an appropriate laboratory setting using
concentrated urine and with the instructions followed exactly by skilled
technicians. At home, with unskilled technicians (us) and urine that may
not be concentrated enough, the sensitivity and accuracy may fall into
the 75 percent range. Using concentrated urine and closely following the
printed instructions are very important. Properly done, the tests are said
to be reliable as early as the first day of a missed period!

A positive test is virtually always correct.

Ultrasound

Everyone who is responsible for the care of pregnant women agrees that
the advent of reliable, high-resolution ultrasound has changed the face of
obstetrics forever. Since its safety during pregnancy is well established, it
has found its way into every conceivable alcove of maternal and fetal
care. You will find an immense section on ultrasound procedures in the
appendix, and it will come up in almost every chapter as we proceed.

For the moment, though, we are presented with one of the first contro-
versies in your prenatal care: Should you have an ultrasound at the beginning of your pregnancy, especially if no problem exists? Should you obtain
a picture just so you know that it is there, a picture that you and he can
look at and maybe put away for some future baby book? Even though a
picture may be worth a thousand words, will your HMO agree?

Well, it's a big and widely opened can of worms at the moment. The
naysayers suggest that ultrasound doesn't contribute sufficient information in a normal pregnancy to make it financially or otherwise worthwhile. They agree with most insurance providers—that it is a waste of
money. The other side (mine) says that an early routine ultrasound:

•absolutely confirms the pregnancy;

•absolutely confirms its location;

•absolutely dates the pregnancy (knowledge that may be invaluable later on); and,

•performed at the proper time, discovers 75 percent of all fetal anomalies.

Current opinion now supports the routine use of ultrasound in early pregnancy. Nevertheless, in today's managed world, your provider may not cover the cost of routine ultrasound.

The Duration of Pregnancy

The duration of pregnancy from fertilization to full-term delivery averages 265 days, but since the day of fertilization is not always known exactly, it is customary to use the first day of the last menstrual period as the marker. That day is more easily pinpointed. You may even have it written down somewhere.

In this book, day 1 is the day of conception and day 265 is the expected date of delivery (EDD). Note, though, that only one mother in 20 delivers on that day; the vast majority deliver within two weeks on either side of it. Some of you may hold on to your precious burden even longer. The longest recorded, thoroughly documented pregnancy was 340 days in duration! This is not likely to happen anymore because we look with suspicion and worry on any pregnancy whose documented length exceeds 42 weeks; we usually do not want them to proceed much longer than that except under very unusual (and clearly explained) circumstances and with exceedingly refined, constant observation and study.

When Will I Deliver? Figuring It Out

A quick way of determining your due date is to add seven days to the first day of your last menstrual period, and then count back three months. For example, let's say your last menstrual period began on March 25. Add seven days to get April 1. Count back three months and—voilà—your due date is January 1 of the next year. If you should deliver a day or so early, you'll get a tax break!

Remember, though, that your due date is just an approximation. If you don't want relatives and friends breathing down your neck at the end, neglect to announce your expected date to anyone, or better still, add a few weeks to it. Otherwise, you will be faced with a steady progression of telephone calls, visits, indiscreet inquiries, secret conferences, and strange looks—all of which may make you wonder whether you and your obstetrician know how to do simple arithmetic.

Telling Your Other Expectant One

At an earlier time in our history, a wife's disclosure of a pregnancy to her husband was a dramatic event equivalent to the great passion play. In our world, there is very little reproductive information that is not instantly available to both partners, and with the advent of early and reasonably accurate home pregnancy testing, Father may be telling Mother the great news if he ends up doing the test.

As our story unfolds, we will draw the expectant father more and more into the relationship that we hope he develops with the child during your pregnancy. We will talk about his relationship with you as well, and about various educational classes and experiences now available that will make him more of a participant in the labor process.

Incidentally, a recent study showed that fully 60 percent of all expectant fathers had some symptoms of pregnancy. This is called the "couvade" syndrome. These poor men may have nausea and vomiting in the mornings, unusual food cravings, headaches, weight increases, and the like. Strangely, or maybe not so strangely, some animal fathers develop the same problems!

Selecting Your Doctor

There has been a dramatic shift in the way medicine is practiced in the few short years since our last edition was published. Managed care is the present medical watchword, and neither you nor your physicians are free to move about in this structured and limiting environment. Thus, you may be told where you will get your obstetrical care, from whom, and what hospital(s) you may go to. The managed care movement, while attempting to control medical costs, has put certain limitations on patient-physician-hospital relationships. It is well for you to find out, in advance of your needs if possible, what your limitations are and whether you may see whom you wish or go to the hospital of your choice. As patient resistance grows, these health plans are becoming somewhat more flexible. But—find out.

Should your options be open, there are some very important matters you should consider when choosing a doctor. Do you want a doctor with a single, partner, or multiple practice? Many obstetricians practice in groups of varying sizes. You may not see the same doctor at each prenatal visit or see the doctor you prefer as often as you would like. On the other hand, 24 hours of each and every day and night at least one member of the group is available. He or she knows you, has your records, and is ready to serve you.

There are advantages to having one obstetrician manage your pregnancy. With one obstetrician, it is easier for support, trust, and understanding to develop between the two of you. Your solo doctor, however, may miss more of your prenatal visits because of labor-room responsibilities and may, for any number of reasons, be away when you deliver. Nevertheless, I practiced alone for many years, and it seemed to work quite well, both for me and for my patients.

Whatever your choice—group or solo—you'll want to find out some things about the style of your physician(s). For instance, if you are planning on prepared childbirth or are interested in a birthing suite or any of a number of new childbirth alternatives, will your physicians support your choice? What is their feeling about pain relief during labor? How do they feel about visitors and family in the labor rooms? What hospitals do they use, and what are the hospital policies that might affect you? For example, most facilities offer their own labor preparation classes in which many questions can be set to rest early on.

Most obstetricians now practicing in the United States have had complete residency training and are certified through comprehensive examination by the American Board of Obstetrics and Gynecology. Each obstetrician must be reexamined and recertified every ten years. Moreover, the overwhelming majority of American obstetricians and gynecologists are members of the American College of Obstetricians and Gynecologists, which has its headquarters in Washington, D.C. This college provides a massive number of postgraduate training programs for its members and also works with great energy, through government and private sources, to promote care for all women—particularly underserved women—in the United States.

Certified obstetricians are available almost everywhere in this country. In some communities, family physicians continue to provide pregnancy care. Clearly, they practice within the limits of their training and, when necessary, refer complicated obstetrical cases for special care. It is worth noting, however, that both obstetricians and family physicians are giving up obstetrics at an alarming rate as malpractice claims escalate. In some states, at least the first $1,000 of each delivery fee goes to support the malpractice process, and it comes from you—not your obstetrician or an insurance company.

In days gone by, women had a very dependent relationship with their obstetrician. Their doctor was, after all, their one source of support through the pain and perils of childbirth and their prime attendant throughout labor. Nowadays, with family-centered pregnancy care and the incredible safety of modern pregnancy, the physician has become more of a provider of services. This new role may be better than the old one, but a certain amount of trust-transference to the doctor you have selected to lead you through this vital experience may be rewarding. For my part, I have no hesitation, and a significant feeling of security, in developing a temporary dependency on and trust in my pilot when I am flying—a dependency that quickly vanishes when we safely touch down. Think about it.

Calling Your Doctor

Under ordinary circumstances, you should generally plan to see your physician shortly after your pregnancy is established by symptoms or by a pregnancy test. "Ordinary circumstances" means that your pregnancy is, as far as you are aware, normal and that you have no disturbing symptoms—such as spotting, cramping, or significant nausea and vomiting. "Ordinary circumstances" also means that you have no prior history of important obstetrical problems and that you have no serious medical conditions that might complicate pregnancy—diabetes, for instance. Under less than ordinary circumstances, you should call your doctor as soon as you even think you may be pregnant and well before any problems develop. See chapter 2 for more details about your first visit.

Sex Determination

Joan or John? Probably no other question is asked of an obstetrician more frequently than what the sex of the unborn baby will be. However, a doctor's guess is just as good as—and no better than—your own. Without special tests, such as amniocentesis, chorion sampling, and sophisticated ultrasound (all of which are detailed in the appendix), no one can predict the sex of an unborn child.

Of course, sex is determined at the moment of conception. The mature female egg contains one sex chromosome, called X. The mature male sperm has a 50–50 chance of containing either an X or a Y chromosome. If an X-bearing sperm unites with an ovum, the child is a girl; if a Y, it's a boy. Since the determination of the sex is dependent upon which type of sperm happens to fertilize the egg, the child's sex is therefore finally and forever determined by the male. Please note, though, that the basic embryonic plan of all mammals of both sexes is apparently feminine and is driven by the powerful X chromosome—of which females have two but need only one in working order to be a complete female. Male development is due to an interruption of the basic X plan by the smaller Y chromosome. Think about that!

Can we make the little one a boy or girl? If we dip into folklore for a moment (and this book often will), throughout history people have made many attempts to preselect or predetermine the sex of an offspring, including reciting certain chants not before or after but *during* sexual intercourse; timing sexual contact in relation to wind direction, rainfall, temperature, or phases of the moon or tides; and eating sweet food to produce girls and bitter food to produce boys (a practice that may have yielded the old "sugar and spice and everything nice" rhyme). In the United States in years gone by, a man hung his pants on the right side of the bed if he wanted a son and on the left if he wanted a daughter—and plopped them on the floor, I guess, if he just wanted to spend the night. These methods are, of course, not exactly reliable in planning the sex distribution of your family. In fact, the only failure-proof folk method of controlling the sex of newborns was to destroy babies of the sex not desired! As cruel as this may seem, various cultures, ranging from the ancient Eskimos to the Maori of New Zealand and the Toda of India, did exactly that. The result was nine living male births for every living female birth! Such unacceptable practices, it is hoped, have long since vanished from the earth—although that may just be wishful thinking.

In fertility study centers today, methods of sperm separation are being improved upon all the time and can now be offered as mechanically or chemically separated X and Y sperm. Such sperm are being used in artificial insemination and in advanced fertilization centers where fertilization is accomplished outside the uterus and the fertilized embryo is then implanted in the uterus. It may be used when there are serious genetic disorders on the sex chromosomes that affect only one sex.

Of course, once your child is conceived, its sex can be accurately determined by a chromosome culture of amniotic fluid, chorionic sampling, or even high-resolution ultrasound (see the appendix).

Here are some surprising facts about the sex ratio at birth that may interest you.

- The percentage of male births is slightly greater than the percentage of female births.

- The percentage of male births rises during and after wars.

- The percentage of female births increases directly with the age of the mother, father, or both.

- The percentage of female births increases with birth rank—that is, first births are more likely than subsequent births to be male.

- A higher percentage of sons are born to couples of greater socioeconomic status.

- The ratio of sons to daughters is higher for couples with a higher sexual intercourse rate.

- The ratio of sons to daughters is slightly lower among blacks than among Caucasians.

- Sex ratio varies with the seasons; in the United States, for instance, the ratio of male to female births is highest in June.

- The ratio of male to female births has been lower after certain natural disasters, such as floods, earthquakes, and epidemics.

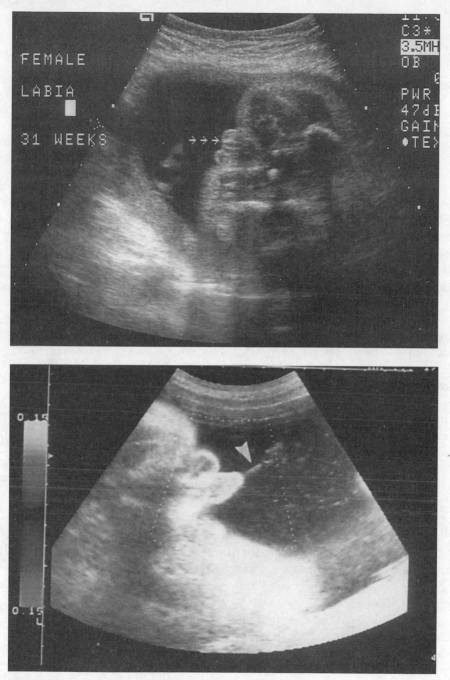

These two pictures demonstrate ultrasound visualization of the reproductive organs. The top picture depicts the female reproductive organs. The lower picture, the male reproductive organs; it shows urination in action. (From *The New England Journal of Medicine*)

Ectopic Pregnancy

Whenever pregnancy occurs in an organ or location outside the uterus, it is termed ectopic. Although this condition would seem to be very unusual, in actuality its incidence is increasing, so that now 1 percent of all pregnancies are ectopic. An important reason for this increase is the exploding incidence of sexually transmitted pelvic infections in young women—disorders that cripple the tubes and arrest ovum passage through them. Most frequently, ectopic pregnancies occur in one fallopian tube or the other, but they are also found in the ovaries and even free in the abdomen. The most unlikely pregnancy of all occurs when the uterus and tubes have been surgically removed by hysterectomy. Under such strange circumstances, we have to assume that a tiny sinus tract persists in the back of the vagina leading to the intra-abdominal cavity, and it is through this that the sperm may migrate and actually fertilize an egg from ovaries that were left behind at the time of hysterectomy. Yes, ovaries left in after a hysterectomy can continue to ovulate; the resultant eggs ordinarily are absorbed without difficulty, just as they are after tubes are tied to produce sterilization.

We are not fully aware of all the circumstances that can lead to ectopic pregnancies. They are most commonly associated, however, with acute and chronic pelvic infections, previous abdominal surgery, endometriosis, previous ectopics, repeated elective abortions, and the use of an intrauterine device (IUD).

Usually ectopic pregnancies end within the first month or two after they have embedded, but the medical literature reports rare cases of pregnancies in the tube, ovary, and even the abdominal cavity that have actually gone to full term and even resulted in a live birth!

The symptoms of an ectopic pregnancy are those of pregnancy, coupled generally with pain in the region where it is embedded. Often the pregnancy, being contained in a sac that cannot expand, as can the uterus, suddenly ruptures. This produces a very acute condition accompanied by severe pain, intra-abdominal bleeding, shock, and collapse.

You should suspect such an abnormal pregnancy if your period is late and you have persistent lower abdominal cramping of a menstrual character (more likely on one side) and episodes of weakness or occasional vaginal spotting.

Thus, if a fertilized egg implants in, say, the left fallopian tube, then besides the usual signs of pregnancy (missed periods, tender breasts, and so on), there will be increasing, left-sided, cramping pain. Note, though, that many other conditions of early *normal* pregnancy produce side pains of varying degrees, ligament pain and corpus luteum pain being two good examples. So don't panic, but do call your doctor.

Once the diagnosis is established, an ectopic pregnancy is usually treated by surgically removing the pregnancy and the affected tubal por-

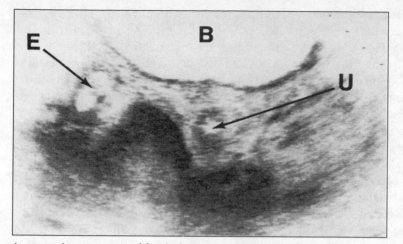

An ectopic pregnancy (E) of about seven weeks' duration and unruptured. The uterus (U) contains a false sac, which can be very misleading. The big white area is a full bladder (B). In this real-time scan, the fetal heart could be seen beating.

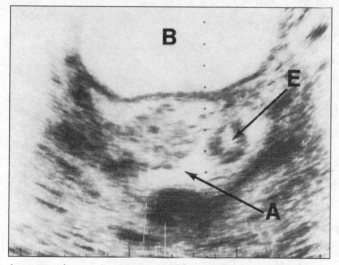

A ruptured ectopic pregnancy (E) with free blood in the abdomen (A). The large white area is a full bladder (B).

tion. This is not a dangerous operation unless, of course, the pregnancy has ruptured from its containing area and there has been a great deal of bleeding and shock. Using certain newer procedures, the surgeon can open the tube, remove the pregnancy, and repair the tube. This procedure, however, depends upon a number of favorable circumstances and is not always possible.

Very recently developed techniques have significantly altered these time-honored surgical approaches. With a high index of suspicion, and using beta HCG blood levels along with transvaginal ultrasound as a guide, it is now possible to locate and diagnose ectopic pregnancies at a very early, unruptured stage. Absolute confirmation may be obtained with a laparoscope. With the diagnosis firmly established, a drug called methotrexate is given. This drug destroys the pregnancy and it disappears. Thus, major surgery and potential tubal destruction are avoided. This drug cannot be used for all ectopics, and its use has to be monitored very carefully to make certain that all pregnancy elements are truly gone.

Although the risk of a recurrent ectopic pregnancy is just around 10 percent, the chances of later having a *normal*-term pregnancy are somewhat reduced. The reason for this disturbing fact is uncertain.

As you can see, it is important that an early ectopic diagnosis be made whenever possible. This is not always simple to do, but again, physicians are being assisted by the beta HCG pregnancy test and by more sophisticated ultrasound procedures and other diagnostic techniques (see the appendix). Moreover, when an early diagnosis is made and confirmed, it is more likely that the newer, simpler management can be used.

A Re-Cap on Ectopic Pregnancy

- **Incidence:** 1 out of every 100 pregnancies.

- **Location:** usually the fallopian tubes; rarely, the ovary or abdomen.

- **Symptoms:** those of pregnancy plus one-sided abdominal pain.

- **Possible complications:** rupturing and severe internal bleeding.

- **Diagnosis:** examination, beta HCG blood test, transvaginal ultrasound, laparoscopy.

- **Treatment:** surgical removal or methotrexate dissolution when possible.

- **Recurrence rate in subsequent pregnancies:** 10 percent.

- **Future normal pregnancy rate:** diminished, but better with the new treatment programs.

Pills, Powders, and Panaceas

Our culture is pill-oriented; we demand pills for everything from looking or feeling bad to smelling bad. Pills are often just adult pacifiers, promoted by a powerful pharmaceutical industry, huckstered by an equally powerful advertising industry, and gobbled up by us in the billions. This phenomenon is problem enough on its own, but in the pregnant community it can become a nightmare in its effect on two people: the host mother and the dependent, developing fetus.

Studies show that pregnant women take an average of 11 over-the-counter drugs during pregnancy—the consequences of which are still largely unknown. Before the thalidomide crisis (which occurred in Europe, not here), the safety of drugs prescribed for pregnant women did not have to be proven. Consequently, little was known about these drugs' potential for fetal harm. Certain medication/pregnancy facts, however, are now made clear by recent research.

- Almost any drug ingested by a pregnant woman, for whatever reason, reaches the bloodstream of her child in a proportional dose *equal* to or *greater* than hers—and within a relatively short period of time.

- This period of time varies from drug to drug, and the relative concentration also varies.

- It was once believed that the larger the molecular structure of a drug, the longer it would take to cross over the placenta; thus, less of the drug would reach the fetus. However, the so-called placental barrier can now be largely considered a myth.

- Babies develop their organ systems and body structure almost completely during the first 12 weeks of pregnancy. At the end of this time, they are very miniature, completely formed humans. For the remaining 28 weeks, these organ systems simply mature and increase in size.

It is clear, then, that the most critical time when structural abnormalities may occur in the developing fetus is during the first 12 weeks. Further, deleterious drugs and diseases work their effects in the various organ systems depending upon when the drug was taken or the disease was contracted. Using thalidomide as an example, if the drug was taken on the 22nd day of the pregnancy, it produced disorders of the upper extremities; taken on the 28th day, disorders of the lower extremities resulted.

It is important to realize that, although development of the organ systems and body structure is generally completed by the 12th week, some drugs and some conditions can affect the developing infant at any and all stages of pregnancy. Lack of proper nourishment, sudden and significant deficits in oxygen, certain types of radiation, and certain maternal habits such as smoking, alcohol consumption, recreational drug use, and certain sexually transmitted infections—all these and many more lifestyle matters can, and do, harm the fetus. We will try and get to them all.

I have before me a vast accumulation of recent literature concerning drugs that can affect mothers and babies during pregnancy. It is not only vast; it is ominous and it is growing, for as you may already know, even "take two aspirins" is no longer considered a safe order. As far as self-medication is concerned, such simple and commonly used medications as aspirin, baking soda, and even some cold preparations are not considered entirely safe insofar as harmful fetal effects are concerned.

As our story unfolds, we will be discussing in greater detail the effects of nicotine, alcohol, cocaine, marijuana, LSD, heroin, and other drugs on the human fetus and on pregnancy. We will see what drugs obstetricians must use during pregnancy, labor, and delivery that may affect you and your baby. And finally, we will list other medications, received from whatever source, and for whatever reason, that are contraindicated in pregnancy. Today there are many frequently used drugs in our households—such as antidepressants, anticonvulsants, diuretics, antibiotics, and pain relievers—that may have adverse effects on the human fetus. We'll get to them.

What must be weighed and considered by you and your doctor first is the benefit-to-risk ratio that applies when using various medications during *your* pregnancy. You should remember *never* to use any medication without consulting your physician. You will soon be aware of the deleterious effects of nicotine, alcohol, and other social drugs upon your pregnancy—and therefore upon your baby—and you must consult your doctor if you think that you cannot avoid their continued use. For the moment, it is reasonable to say that no drug given in the first weeks of pregnancy can be considered safe, unless your doctor gives it the thumbs-up—calcium supplements might be an example.

In addition, some women's work puts them into areas that expose them to certain chemicals, vapors, or radioactive elements, making it necessary for them to consider retirement as soon as pregnancy is determined. This is covered on page 56.

What is important for you to remember, then, is to take no medication during your pregnancy that is not prescribed by your doctor. Make sure that any other physician you consult for any reason is made aware of your pregnancy, if it is not visibly clear, and that your obstetrician is informed about and concurs with any medications or treatments proposed for you.

All prescription drugs are listed in the *PDR* (*Physician's Desk Reference*), a large book published annually and updated quarterly. Each drug has a pregnancy rating—A to X—with A being safe and X forbidden. Most drugs are rated C—the pregnancy effect in humans is unknown, unproven, or uncertain. If you do not wish to ask your doctor about a certain agent, the *PDR* can be found in most public libraries or on the Internet. Try your doctor first.

Let's now revisit and summarize these pregnancy problems that we have been looking at. Although they will all be dealt with in much greater detail later in the book, they are important enough to reemphasize at this early point. Avoid, then:

- **Any drug for whatever reason.** Unless a drug is cleared by the doctor responsible for you during your pregnancy, avoid all drugs. This includes over-the-counter nonprescription drugs—even aspirin. Record in this book any drug that you may have taken inadvertently before your pregnancy was diagnosed. Chapter 4 points out the safety of various prescription and nonprescription drugs during your pregnancy.

- **Smoking.** The 27,000 chemical insults a fetus receives with each of its mother's inhalations during a tobacco pregnancy may mark it forever as slow to grow and slow to learn. The dangerous effects of tobacco on your fetus are reviewed in chapter 3.

- **Alcohol.** You should not drink while pregnant. The consumption of alcohol during pregnancy is directly related to the increasing incidence of very significant fetal disorders. The dangerous effects of alcohol on your fetus are explained in chapter 3.

- **Violent physical activity.** Most exercise and sports are fine, but exhausting, stressful physical competition directs more blood to skeletal muscles to sustain performance. Visceral organ centers are deprived of blood, including the uterus. Miscarriage or fetal damage is therefore more likely. Safe sports and exercises are discussed in chapter 2.

- **Accidents.** Automobile accidents in particular are the leading cause of maternal (and thus fetal) deaths. Seat belts are now mandatory almost everywhere and, properly used, pose no risk to your intrauterine cargo. Similarly, air bags will protect all but the shortest mothers and their unborn babies. While there is great turmoil over air bags at present, the medical profession's consensus is *do not disconnect*.

- **Sexually transmitted diseases.** Many sexually transmitted diseases have severe, even fatal, fetal complications. AIDS has become a leading killer of women of childbearing age—and their babies. These diseases are covered in detail in chapter 4.

- **Malnutrition.** Often related to dietary habits rather than to poverty, malnutrition is a leading cause of prematurity and the number-one cause of infant mortality and morbidity in the United States!

- **Certain paints.** Please be cautious and careful when using oils and other paints containing barium, cadmium, or lead—for whatever home-repair or hobby purpose. Wash your hands thoroughly after use. Avoid the inadvertent ingestion and inhalation of house paints, including latex paints that contain lead or mercury (a preservative). Use spray paints only in a well-ventilated area; the propellants are toxic. These dangers are explained in more detail in chapter 3.

- **Pets, wild animals, and birds.** Avoid all strange cats and wild animals. These animals may carry diseases that could adversely affect your pregnancy. These dangers are discussed in more detail in chapters 4 and 6.

Now, let's look hard at this whole list. These dangers are all nonobstetrical factors that interfere with the normal events of pregnancy. They vastly outweigh any obstetrical problems that you are likely to face, and for the most part, they are within your control. Good health is mainly good education—and good sense.

"Do as I Say"

Compliance ("do as I say") is, in medicine, a sensitive and vastly important subject that we need to look at for a minute. It has nothing to do with "control or surrender." It has to do with responsibility. Many studies indicate clearly that medicines prescribed by physicians are not taken by their patients and that instructions given are not regularly followed. Such failure to comply with what we have been told and what we know is right involves all aspects of our lives (the use of seat belts and baby seats in automobiles, for instance), and all of us are guilty, doctors included. Usually compliance with medical instructions is an individual matter that each of us can manage at a personal level, taking or disregarding the advice presented to us. Pregnancy is another matter—a loaded matter. For we are now dealing with the health and welfare of a helpless, dependent, and very, very vulnerable human being. So give your baby your best shot: follow your doctor's advice.

Some Pregnant Pauses

- In 1522, the first doctor who tried to get into a delivery chamber to learn more about the process, a man named Von Wert, dressed himself in women's clothes. He was discovered and burned to death.

•In 1847, Ignaz Semmelweis, the first doctor to prove that childbirth fever—a major cause of maternal death—is contagious, lost his hospital appointment in Vienna, was ridiculed out of his practice by his colleagues, and committed suicide.

•In 1880, James P. White, the first doctor to teach obstetrics to other doctors in the United States (in Buffalo, New York), was hounded into obscurity.

•The first female physician was an Egyptian. Peseshet, who was identified by many important titles, including "Overseer of Women Physicians," was discovered when excavation of the tomb of Akhet-Hetep at Giza revealed a monument dedicated to her. She is probably the world's earliest-known woman physician. She practiced at the time of the building of the great pyramids in Egypt, about 2500 B.C. (Incidentally, the first and only woman pharaoh, Hatshepsut, ruled Egypt some 1,000 years later—after 2,000 years of male pharaohs.)

•As we shall see later, the history of cesarean sections is not a robust, healthy chapter in the annals of medicine. Early on, survivors— either mother or babe—were the marked exception. After a massive search of historical literature, excluding antiquity and legends, the very first recorded cesarean section in which the mother survived that I can find occurred in 1739—some 260 years ago. The surviving mother was named Alice O'Neal. Her babe, sadly, did not survive. The operating surgeon? Mary Dunally, a midwife!

•There are, at this time, about 58 million American women of childbearing age—15 to 44 years. Here is their track record:
   Some 35 million use some form of contraception, including tubal ligation.
   Over 5 million have infertility problems, and 20 percent of those women seek help each year.
   About 6 million pregnancies occur each year, and at least 15 percent of the established pregnancies miscarry—but undoubtedly many more are lost before pregnancy is even considered, let alone established.
   About 1.6 million pregnancies will terminate by induced abortion.
   All but 1.2 percent of the live births will take place in a hospital or birthing center, and 95.7 percent of those deliveries will be managed by doctors.

•The upper age limit of pregnancy is gradually being extended further into senior years as childbearing is delayed and fertility programs are extended.

Diary

My First Month

Last period_____

Symptoms_____

_____

_____

Bleeding_____

_____

_____

Illness_____

_____

_____

Medications_____

_____

What's going on in the world?_____

_____

_____

_____

What's going on in my life?_____

_____

_____

_____

My thoughts and feelings_____

_____

_____

_____

Doctor's appointment_____

_____

_____

Questions to ask_____

_____

_____

_____

_____

_____

_____

_____

_____

_____

_____

_____

_____

_____

_____

_____

_____

_____

_____

_____

_____

_____

_____

_____

_____

_____

Two

My Second Lunar Month

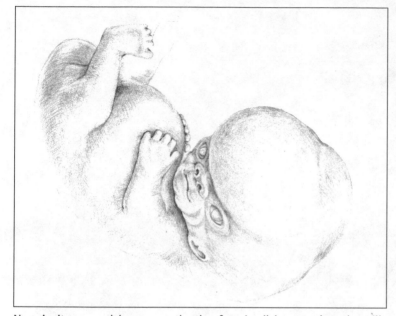

Now in its second lunar month, the fetus' tail is gone but the gills linger on. They will soon wither away, however, as internal organ systems continue their rapid establishment. The fetal heart—still a simple tube—is beating, and has been since 21 days after conception (you would then be but one week overdue!), a few days before it can be visualized by the most advanced ultrasound. A circulatory system is developing along with limbs and finger and toe buds. It is less than an inch long (2.4 centimeters) and has yet to move.

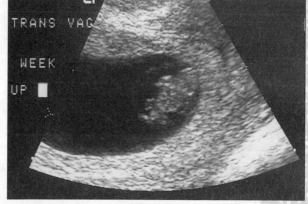

On trans-vaginal ultra-sound, this little embryo can now be seen enclosed in its black-appearing amniotic sac.

Having now missed your second period and having suffered one or more of the monumental initial maladies that no one else believes, you are convinced of what is going on and feel that it is time to convince the world, your doctor, and your significant other of the same thing. This is about the time that most expectant mothers call their obstetrician for the first appointment—and rightly so, because prior to this time it is usually difficult to determine for sure, without those special tests, whether pregnancy exists. Of course, there are exceptions to this rule, and if any of the following abnormal conditions exists, you should consult your doctor immediately, no matter how far along you consider yourself to be:

- You are involved in an extensive infertility program.

- You have a history of repeated miscarriages.

- You are experiencing severe lower abdominal cramping.

- You have a history of ectopic pregnancy.

- You are experiencing vaginal bleeding.

- You are suffering from severe nausea or vomiting.

No matter what stage of pregnancy you believe that you are in, any of these conditions requires immediate consultation with your doctor.

First Visit to Your Doctor

The first time you visit your obstetrician, a typical series of events will most likely occur. Your medical history will be taken. Sometimes this history is very detailed, and you may be asked to fill in this form yourself. It may contain more than 100 questions related to your present health, past health, any previous surgery or serious illnesses you have had, any medications you may now be taking or may have taken in the past few months, your family history, genetic history, even your emotional attitude toward your pregnancy.

Although these questions may seem unusually detailed, they are of significant value because your doctor must know as much as possible about you in order to manage your pregnancy properly. Moreover, answering these questions may refresh your memory and bring forward some significant medical problems that you had forgotten. Example: a question may remind you that you did indeed have a fever and some swollen glands after a cat scratch years ago. That could be important information.

One of the initial questions your obstetrician or an associate will ask you is when you think your last period might have taken place. From what you have already read, you may now understand how important that date can be. Try to have the correct date available when that question comes up.

Some women keep no record of their cyclical menstrual events, preferring to relate them to some social, political, sporting, or catastrophic event that took place about the same time. Unfortunately your doctor does not always have ready access to your personal frame of reference, and it may be asking a lot of him or her to recall an event important to you alone. So don't tell your doctor that your last period was the day before Oprah won her legal battle with the beef industry!

Some very well-organized women keep their menstrual records at hand somewhere in their checkbook, on a calendar, or scribbled on an old parking ticket, a grocery slip, a failed lottery stub, or some other wonderfully accessible place. No matter how you keep track of your cycles, it would be to your advantage to have the date of the first day of your last menstrual cycle ready when you arrive for your first appointment.

You may take comfort in learning that many of the doctors whom I have delivered over the years had no better knowledge of their last menstrual period than anyone else!

At your first visit, you will also have a physical examination. The regular, routine physical exam includes evaluation of your whole body as well as a detailed pelvic exam. If your history reveals any significant physical or anatomical problems, special attention is given to those areas at this time. The pelvic examination determines, insofar as possible, the presence of pregnancy, its location and duration, and whether there are any accompanying pelvic diseases or disorders. The doctor is also assessing your bony pelvic structure.

Blood tests will be given, and certain other laboratory work will be done. Blood tests are done to determine:

- your hemoglobin level and other routine blood counts

- your blood type and Rh factor

- the presence of any circulating immune antibodies in your system that might affect pregnancy—Rh antibodies, for instance

- your immunity to German measles (rubella) and toxoplasmosis (cat fever)

A test for syphilis is still mandatory in most states. As for AIDS, while desirable, a test is neither widely accepted yet nor mandatory. Also not yet mandatory in most areas is a test for hepatitis B, although it may soon become so designated and your own doctor may test for it.

Further laboratory work at this time usually includes a urinalysis (sometimes even a urine culture may be routinely done), and a Papanicolaou (Pap) smear, for routine detection of cervical cancer. Moreover, early-pregnancy screening for sexually transmitted diseases other than syphilis and AIDS is becoming much more common as the incidence of sexually transmitted diseases soars. Chlamydia and gonor-rhea are the two most commonly sought out. Note also that newer blood tests and procedures are commonly and constantly being added to the list of determinations made at both the initial and subsequent visits. Also, certain blood tests are performed as your pregnancy advances. Thus, maternal serum alpha-fetoprotein (MSAFP) blood screening will be done for Down's syndrome detection between your 15th and 18th week. At the same time, two other blood tests may be done (HCG—remember?— and free estriol) in order to strengthen a Down's diagnosis. Additionally, it has recently been suggested that genetic blood testing for cystic fibrosis be offered in all pregnancies. Around the 28th week of pregnancy, a blood sugar test is usually done to observe for potential gestational dia-betes. If your blood sugar is abnormal, further in-depth sugar studies will be done. And so it goes—you may begin to wonder if any of your own blood remains!

We have already noted that an ultrasound may be performed early in your pregnancy and have given you the reasoning behind it. This proce-dure may not be done at your first visit, since it will be more meaningful a few weeks further on.

Eventually, all this mental and physical probing will end, you will be dressed and sitting up, and you and your doctor will have a talk in which you will be given detailed advice—or this book containing such advice. Necessary prenatal vitamin-mineral supplements will be prescribed, questions will be answered, money will be brought up and explained (although this may take place later with an office assistant), and subse-quent appointments will be made (again, by someone else).

After all this, you may feel by the time you leave the doctor's office that you have forgotten your due date, your own and your doctor's names, and whether or not you put all your clothes back on—and in proper order! When you settle down, be sure to record your doctor's reg-ular office phone number and emergency number on the telephone list provided at the beginning of this book. Then go home, sit down, and have a drink—but not alcohol.

Subsequent Visits

If your pregnancy is quite normal, your return visits to your obstetrician start out at monthly intervals and become progressively more frequent as time goes on. Such visits give your doctor ample opportunity to follow your progress and, if your doctor practices alone, for you both to develop a feeling of mutual trust and confidence. In group practices, you will become familiar with each one in the gang and will see a familiar face when you come to labor and delivery.

Each time you return, you will follow a routine catechism of procedures interspersed with special procedures that we will learn about as we move forward in our journey. Here are some of the routine procedures:

- You will be weighed. Yuck!

- Your blood pressure will be checked.

- Your urine will be tested for sugar, protein, evidence of infection, and more.

- As soon as it is useful, examination of the abdomen will be done to measure uterine growth as it rises into the abdomen.

- Generally by the third month—or shortly thereafter—a fetoscope listening device placed upon your lower abdomen will allow you, your doctor, and anyone else in the room to hear your infant's heartbeat—sometimes even its excursions around its intrauterine home.

- Your extremities will be checked for edema (swelling).

- You will be asked to point out any problem areas that need evaluation.

Special procedures will be done—or ordered—as indicated as your pregnancy progresses. We will look at all of these in order.

Usually you will then get a chance to talk things over—sitting up—with your doctor. Sometimes your visit may be conducted by a nurse-practitioner or a midwife employed by your doctor(s). This may be more rewarding!

Use the section at the end of each chapter to record any problems or questions you want to deal with during your visits. Although pelvic examinations are generally omitted from routine repeat visits, one will be done if you have any unusual symptoms such as local irritation, spotting, or other unusual discharges. Toward the end of pregnancy, you will again be favored with internal pelvic examinations to assess the condition of your cervix, find the position of your baby, and reevaluate your pelvic measurements. Very slight spotting may follow these quite safe internal examinations for 24 hours or so and are not a worry.

Discomforts in Early Pregnancy

There can be several sorts of maladies or discomforts early on to remind you that you are with child. They include:

- •morning sickness

- •mouth watering

- •lower abdominal discomfort

- •breast tenderness

- •bladder problems

- •weariness, fainting, and headaches

These discomforts are usually not serious but, under certain circumstances, may become so. We shall see.

Morning Sickness

Most often, morning sickness (nausea and vomiting) is a problem confined to the first three months of pregnancy. You have a 50–50 chance of being so affected, and even if you are, you may not be bothered very much, particularly if you follow the advice coming up. In rare cases, a woman may continue to be nauseated throughout her pregnancy, but if nausea does persist, something else is usually amiss and the doctor will find it.

No one has the complete answer as to why nausea and vomiting are visitors in so many early pregnancies—but it is a real, nonimaginary problem.

To treat morning nausea:

- •Avoid fried, fatty, or greasy foods; highly seasoned foods (Mexican and Italian dishes, barbecue, sausage, luncheon meat, ham, and so on); rich foods (such as pastries, pies, cakes). What's left? Seemingly precious little—but more than enough.

- •Prepare low-fat meat, poultry, and fish by roasting, baking, or grilling. Vegetables that have been steamed, roasted, or boiled will also do just fine. So will simple desserts and fresh fruits. Bland carbohydrates such as rice, pasta, couscous, polenta, and other cereals and grains are excellent sources of nourishment now—and at anytime. They can be adorned in many succulent ways without hot seasoning.

•Eat frequently. Avoid big meals, and divide your daily rations into multiple small feedings that you take every hour or two insofar as possible. Try to leave food at your bedside so that when you get up at night for your bathroom sojourns, you can nibble on a little something, like crackers, a plain cookie, or a piece of fruit. Don't follow this part of the plan if you have the gastroesophageal reflux (GERD) disorder—but if you do, you should already know it and be under appropriate treatment.

•Always try to eat before you get up in the morning and before you go to bed at night (again, except for GERD)—not much, but some. If you work, carry crackers, cookies, quartered sandwiches, fruit, celery sticks, and carrot sticks with you.

•If you eat out, avoid large meals and fast-food restaurants—at this time in your life, fast foods mean fast in, fast down, fast up, and fast out. Your basic goal is never to let your stomach get empty—or too full.

•Avoid medications for the control of nausea and vomiting—unless prescribed by your doctor. Vitamin B_6 (50 milligrams per tablet), which is not a medicine but rather a high dose of a known vitamin, is sometimes used to manage morning sickness, but even it has been avoided by some. The early months of pregnancy are such a sensitive time that physicians are loath to order, and mothers are loath to take anything, that might conceivably alter the normal development of a child—despite the fact that there are known safe medications for this time period.

•Consider taking a short leave of absence if your work requires a great deal of concentration or manual skills and if your nausea is severe. You will soon be feeling better and will want to continue your work. If, on the other hand, you have a job with a flexible work pattern, try to keep going. This is important advice at a time when you could stay home and feel very sorry for yourself, which is never good medicine.

•Be aware that some very, very few individuals become sick enough from constant vomiting to necessitate a trip to the hospital. This is particularly important if there has been enough fluid loss to produce dehydration and to disturb systemic electrolyte balance. Hospital treatment involves intravenous replacement of fluids, food, and electrolytes, and sometimes the use of certain drugs. You and your doctor would discuss the benefit-risk ratio. Generally, the disorder risk is severe enough that something must be done, and almost anything beats persistent dehydration and starvation.

• Report any blood that you observe in what you throw up. Very occasionally, persistent vomiting produces a little blood, generally because the stomach lining is irritated. It is usually not harmful or dangerous but should be reported. Pretty soon the good times will roll again!

Cramps

Slight menstrual cramps are apt to occur, particularly at the time you are missing a period. Your uterus questions the new passenger that is stretching its walls, and so it cramps back ever so lightly. These pains may last a day or two but are very moderate in nature. They may recur from time to time but never with increasing discomfort. If the cramping should become severe or be associated with any spotting whatsoever, your doctor should be called at once, as this is an abnormal sign and needs some management.

Ligament Pain

Very commonly in the early months of pregnancy, your uterus, as it grows, turns slightly to one side or the other—more often to the right. Such twisting produces a pulling pain, usually in the lower right side of the abdomen. You will notice it most frequently when you get up quickly or turn sharply from one side to the other, and you may feel it on both sides. This pain, present only in the early months of pregnancy, is only nagging in nature and of no real significance. Any other pain in the lower abdomen or pain that is crippling should be reported.

Other Pain

The corpus luteum cyst on one ovary or the other may cause some pain on the side where it resides. This cyst, you remember, forms at the spot on your ovary where ovulation took place. It supplies increasing amounts of progesterone for the first three months of your pregnancy, thereafter being supplanted in this task by the infant's placenta. Progesterone is the hormone without which a pregnancy cannot be maintained. Miscarriage or labor always follows its withdrawal.

Sometimes in the early months this very normal and important cyst can cause pain where it resides—pain that may be confused with more serious conditions. Careful examinations or ultrasound can delineate the source of such pain, and can be very reassuring.

Mouth Watering

Rarely, an increase in the flow of saliva (ptyalism) is noted for the first few months. Again, the cause of this minor condition is unknown. There are no treatments that alter it, so that leaves us with two solutions: either to swallow down the saliva or to spit it out. Neither solution is entirely agreeable, but there is nothing else to offer.

Breasts

The breasts' first reason for being is to suckle the newborn. Thus, very early in pregnancy, stimulated by fertilization, the breasts become congested and tender. Though you may have noticed in the past that your breasts were uncomfortable just before menstruation, the fullness and discomfort that occur in early pregnancy are usually somewhat greater. This increased congestion is due to the final development of the breasts' glandular milk-secreting system. All of a sudden, it is distressing for you to jog, ride in a jeep, play tennis, take a shower, sleep on your stomach, make love, make haste, or do anything that moves your body faster or higher or lower or quicker than your breasts.

Your breasts will be more comfortable when supported with a well-fitting bra but should never be bound in any way. You may even find it a relief to wear your bra while you are sleeping. If you do not regularly wear a bra, your discomfort may be somewhat greater and the milk precursor—colostrum—may stain your garments.

Breasts begin their growth and glandular development in early pregnancy, more rapidly during the first few months and then continuing at a much slower rate. You may require a larger cup as pregnancy advances. Very rapid breast growth may be accompanied by stretch marks (striae) in the skin. Striae may be minimized somewhat by using breast support, avoiding excessive weight gain, and massaging your breasts each night with a lanolin-based skin cream.

Sometime during pregnancy—usually early on—a clear secretion may be noted coming from your nipples. This, again, is colostrum, the fore-runner of true milk, which does not appear until after you deliver. The secretion of colostrum may increase during lovemaking. No real problem. Finally, alas, as a result of all the pregnancy changes, your breast size may increase or decrease significantly and forever, and I cannot explain why this happens. But it does.

Incidentally, the congestion of your breast tissue at this time may produce areas that seem to be lumps or cysts. Your doctor will be happy to check these areas if reminded during a visit. Mammograms taken during pregnancy are perfectly safe when you are properly shielded and should not be avoided if there is a compelling reason. However, because of the breast congestion, they may be more difficult to interpret.

Bladder

Position means a lot in life, and it is the unfortunate position of your bladder to lie in front of your uterus. During pregnancy, uterine congestion and swelling put pressure on its watery neighbor, which in turn puts pressure on you. Very early in your pregnancy, then, you may find that a good deal of your life is spent going to and coming from the bathroom. This bladder pressure is somewhat overcome in the middle months of pregnancy as the uterus rises, but later, as the baby's head settles down into the pelvis toward full term, your bladder once again fills at shorter intervals. Like a car with a small gas tank, your excursions are limited.

Women's bladders are connected to the outside world by a very short tube called the urethra. When the urethra is not being used, it is kept closed by a series of muscles that you learned, long ago, to control voluntarily, and that you are shortly going to be teaching that individual in your tummy to control, if you ever want to get out of changing diapers. As pregnancy advances, a good deal of pressure is put on the urethra, and sometimes voluntary muscular control of urination is lost, particularly when you sneeze, lift things, cough, giggle, or shout. This "incontinence" tends to disappear after delivery, although total control may never be quite the same again because of stretched muscles.

Bladder Infections

For a number of reasons, the bladder and, higher up, the kidneys are more susceptible to infection during pregnancy. The symptoms of lower urinary tract infection (cystitis or bladder infection) include frequent and painful urination, with a feeling of incomplete bladder emptying. Occasionally there may even be blood present and visible in the urine.

On the other hand, an upper urinary tract infection (pyelitis or kidney infection) produces many of the symptoms of a lower tract infection plus chills, fever, pain high in the back on one or both sides, along with feelings of acute illness. It is quite possible to have cystitis without pyelitis. You should report any of these abnormal symptoms immediately. Sexual activity will somewhat increase your chances of urinary tract infections at this time—particularly if prolonged, or if locally heavy and active physical events are part of your fore, after, and during play. Your mate's body—particularly his hands, mouth, and genitals—should be very clean. Your bladder should be empty at the beginning and emptied at the end—if possible—and your local hygiene should be the best. You cannot douche or use powders. More on all this later. Just protect your urinary system. Drink.

Yes. Drinking plenty of fluids during pregnancy will help prevent your urine from becoming too concentrated. So drink anything that isn't intoxicating, habit-forming, or polluted. Cranberry juice provides water and further provides some protection against cystitis. Nowhere is the maxim of eight daily glasses of water more valuable than here. Drinking water will not increase your swelling (edema) while you are pregnant—regardless of what you hear. An adequate water intake will actually decrease your swelling.

After you deliver, there may be a number of temporary bladder problems, and we will talk about them when that time comes. Right now, your only goal is to keep the system moving and the channels clear and flowing!

Weariness, Fainting, and Headaches

It's a hot Monday morning, and you are already late for work—work that happens to take place on the 80th floor of a glass tower somewhere downtown. The bus was bad enough, but now you are in a hot, stuffy, crowded elevator—which turns out not to be an express—you should have had breakfast but you were too late, and the guy crowding closest to you should not have had breakfast, or a cigar, but a shower . . . so at about floor 63, your body has had enough and you fall down. There is no place for you to fall in this steamy crowd, so until the elevator stops at the 80th floor, and the doors open, only then can you fall down and out—out of the elevator and out of reality. Small wonder!

Because your blood pressure is low and unstable during early pregnancy, incidents like this are quite common. You faint because, quite literally, your brain is not getting enough blood and, therefore, not enough oxygen. The instability of your blood pressure produces other common symptoms at this time, such as weariness, dizzy spells, and, in some cases, constant dull headaches. Weariness or tiredness is probably the most common of all these complaints. If you work away from home, it is all you can do to struggle home before collapsing. If housework is your lot, you are likely to let a layer of dust settle over the house while you hibernate on the sofa. It is important to know that if you do faint—anywhere—you must be placed lying on one side or the other, or, if you are just woozy, that you sit in a chair and bend your head forward as far as possible. Get up from either position very slowly and, once up, keep going.

It is important to remember that dizziness and the tendency to faint are most likely to occur when you first get up, especially if you get up too

quickly, if you stand or sit too long in one position, or if you are some-
place—like that miserable elevator—that is warm and overcrowded and
you begin to feel boxed in. Try your best to avoid these situations.
Theaters, malls, churches, elevators, buses—anywhere crowded—all are
waiting to get you. You have to get up and get going sooner or later, but
be careful how and where you do it. And keep moving! Keep moving,
that is, unless you feel dizzy again!

Headaches, if they occur, are usually dull and throbbing and are more
likely to be constant during the day but to disappear at night—and to
disappear completely before midpregnancy. Don't take any medication
for these headaches without consulting your doctor.

It may be tempting to quit work when you feel so tired, particularly if
nausea and headaches also accompany your blood pressure instability.
Again, that is a decision you must make based upon some of the variables mentioned earlier about work.

Your social activities should be curtailed when they are not enjoyable
or when they keep you on your feet too long. It is important for your significant other to understand the way you feel at this time and to know
that it is temporary.

There are a number of other, much more serious headaches that may
come along later on. Migraines may flare up, and pregnancy-induced
hypertension also has its own brand of headache that serves as a warning
that all is not well. We will see about these as we progress.

Prone Pressure Syndrome

Though this condition generally involves later pregnancy, we will look
at it here because it also has to do with blood pressure instability.
When your unborn babe is bigger and you lie flat on your back, the
pressure against the major blood vessels and nerves running along your
backbone can produce a sudden and dramatic drop in blood pressure.
This prone pressure syndrome is more likely to occur when you are
lying down somewhere that's rather confining and you have to be still
for a while. Thus, a common place for it to present itself is in your doctor's office, while you wait on your back in the examining room for
him or her to come in and see you. You suddenly begin to feel hot,
sticky, clammy, uncomfortable, ready to faint, and generally very
unhappy with your environment. If this happens, turn immediately
onto either side, but preferably onto your left side, since on that side
maximum pressure is taken off the major blood vessels. Your symptoms will disappear very quickly. The most important thing to remember is this: *Do not, under any circumstances, try to get up.* Wait until
you have been on one side or the other long enough to feel well and stable. Even then, get up slowly, with great care and with a support person
present.

Unusual Food Cravings

Why you should suddenly crave kumquats in the middle of the night and in the dead of winter is hard to understand, but unusual food cravings are common in early pregnancy. You may give in to these wild desires unless they include foods that will increase your tendency to nausea or unless you crave a substance (and this is very rare) that is not a food. Strangely enough, some women experience cravings (called pica) for chalk, clay, coal, cloth, cork, turpentine, and petroleum jelly, among other things. These substances are no worse than some fast foods offered today, but leave them be!

Emotions in Pregnancy

It's midnight, and you have slept (if you want to call it that) for two hours. Now you're wide awake. After going to the bathroom, you turn on the late-late show—*Casablanca,* starring Humphrey Bogart and Ingrid Bergman. You look over at your mate snoring happily, with his foot between you and Bogart's ear. He never needs to get up to go to the john (your mate, not Bogie). He needs his adenoids out, though! You wonder how much that would cost. And now, damn it, Ingrid is going to make the same stupid mistake that she has made the last 50 times you have seen the picture. She is going to get on the plane with that Dutchman!

While your mind is running on like this, all of a sudden, for no apparent reason, you begin to cry, to weep, and to wail. The snoring stops. He wakes up. Bedlam. "What's wrong? What have I done? Call the doctor. Get something to eat. Go to the bathroom. Watch TV. Do anything, but stop crying!" And so is ushered in a new and slightly disturbing companion of early pregnancy, "the blues."

Women are not likely to escape episodes of emotional storms during pregnancy. Most of these storms consist of depressive interludes that come and go, usually in the early months and usually without any apparent cause. So when you have the blues and dissolve into tears and can't understand why, don't worry, and don't try to figure it out. It soon passes. And *he* will recover, too.

Medication is not necessary to control this minor depression or any of the other transient emotional reactions that occur during pregnancy. Generally, though, a serious preexisting emotional problem that already requires regular medication must be individually dealt with by you and your doctor. Medication, particularly in the early months, is, as you already know, best avoided. On the other hand, understanding and tolerance by all who are involved—or who think they are involved—is most important.

As pregnancy draws toward its climax, it is not unnatural for you to become somewhat apprehensive about the outcome for yourself and your baby. You may fear that the baby will be disfigured or deformed or, worst of all, will not survive. Even though you attend reassuring childbirth classes, you may still be apprehensive about the outcome of your labor and delivery. Further, you may fear that your relationship with your mate will be jeopardized, and on and on.

You would be a most unusual person if you did not entertain these fears occasionally and even have some nightmares about them. Moreover, physical discomfort and insomnia, which occur at this late time, plus any underlying problems at home tend to add to your anxieties. Discussion of the problems with your doctor may help. Prenatal courses, too, help relieve your mind about many of the tales you may have heard or any misconceptions you may have concerning pregnancy, labor, and delivery. Avoiding the advice and stories of well-meaning but misguided friends and relatives is probably the most important thing you can do. This is important to know now so that these things won't haunt you as your pregnancy moves forward.

Postpartum Depression

You are probably aware that very shortly after delivery, "baby blues" may occur. This emotional problem generally begins the second or third day after delivery and is characterized by depression, crying spells, a feeling of inadequacy, ambivalence toward your baby and mate, and certain fears. This depression, like that of early pregnancy, is not unusual and, most often, is *temporary* in the vast majority of pregnancies. Usually it disappears just as suddenly as it appeared. However, it very rarely can become a most serious emotional problem and require expert attention from a mental health care provider. Toward the end of this book is an expanded overview of this problem. In the meantime, just remember that serious postpartum depression is rare and that you should not anticipate it or burden yourself with thoughts about it. You've got enough on your plate already!

The most important thing that you and your beloved can do to promote an emotionally healthy pregnancy is to work out, insofar as you can, any tensions in your household. As a matter of fact, this is important not only during pregnancy but for all your life together. Problems between the two of you must be brought out into the open and discussed, vocalized, explored, discussed again, and settled. Some help is needed if a basic issue or problem remains unsettled for any length of time. The development of a prolonged communication barrier between you two is the death knell of a relationship. Your mate is a shareholder, not a perpetrator. You are a shareholder, not a carrier. Don't divide while you are multiplying.

Personal Hygiene

Unless you have some pretty unusual health habits, there are only a few alterations in your personal hygiene to consider while you are pregnant. If you have any particular complication that might interfere with your ordinary hygienic routine, the doctor will provide you with specific instructions to cover that situation.

Pregnancy regularly induces some physiological changes that can interfere with or alter your personal grooming habits. These include:

- •increased perspiration

- •increased body secretions

- •rapid skin stretching

- •altered complexion and skin characteristics

- •increased difficulty in reaching and even seeing some body parts!

Bathing and Showering

You may bathe and shower as frequently as you wish, and you may continue bathing as long as you are able to ease your body safely into the tub. Pregnant women were advised years ago to discontinue tub bathing six weeks prior to their date of delivery. No one knows why they were told this, but it was a monstrous instruction. The only real risk involved is getting into and out of the tub, and since you are not very agile in the last few months, do be careful. There is no need to stop tub-bathing—unless you just prefer showering. However, long hot tub baths—like hot-tub and sauna sojourns—are potentially harmful to your little one, as we will see in a moment.

You may take stall showers whenever you wish, and for as long as you wish, but because of mechanical considerations, showering in a tub is dangerous, particularly in late pregnancy. At that time your balance becomes increasingly less secure, and a slippery sloppy tub is much more difficult to negotiate. Thus, showering in a tub during late pregnancy should be avoided if at all possible. If you have no alternative, be sure to use a suction mat on the tub floor and to have something firm to grasp while getting in and out.

After bathing or showering, you may wish to lubricate your body with a skin cream containing lanolin, particularly if you live in a cold, dry climate or if you already have problems with dry stretched skin. Pay particular attention to your abdomen and breasts, since these areas are where the lines of pregnancy (striae) are most likely to appear. Such lines can be minimized by keeping your skin well lubricated.

Hot Tubs and Saunas

There is *very strong* evidence that hot tubs are not safe during pregnancy, because significant elevations of body temperature, as such bathing produces, can have harmful fetal effects. The same is apparently true for saunas. Moreover, most private hot tubs are not very sanitary; they can harbor harmful bacteria. Public spa facilities are required to keep the water in their saunas and tubs relatively sterile. However, recent evidence shows that plastic surfaces such as the benches used in these areas can culture positively for viruses, including the herpes virus. Further, a recent outbreak of Legionnaires' disease has been traced to a public, power-circulating hot tub. So be careful. The Romans might have had the right idea for their times—but not for ours.

If you can avoid all of these risk situations, then you may certainly indulge in bubble, oil, mud, Japanese, mineral, milk, seaweed, or champagne baths as time and money permit! Just be sure to keep clean and cool. Avoid any prolonged body heat exposure.

Douching

During pregnancy, normal vaginal secretions often increase because of the marked local congestion. Such secretions are generally white and should not be offensive or cause any irritation or itching. It is important to note, though, that certain vaginal infections are also common at this time and may produce a discharge that is offensive or irritating, or both (see pages 104–107).

Vaginal douching, however, is unwise during pregnancy—even dangerous. The cervix is softening and may be slowly thinning and opening somewhat. Thus, the douche nozzle or some of the douche fluid may get into the uterine cavity, with potentially disastrous results.

Therefore, physicians regularly advise against this very personal hygienic practice. If you have strong feelings about it, you certainly must consult with your obstetrician and get his or her advice about douching. Most certainly, however, your doctor will be opposed to it.

Your Hair

Fools rush in where hairdressers fear to tread—but here goes.

In addition to shampooing, you may continue to perm, curl, rat, mousse, blow-dry, and otherwise manipulate your hair, with this important limitation: Avoid any dyes during pregnancy or, for that matter, any chemicals that remain on your hair or scalp for any length of time. This ban does not include modest amounts of hair-setting spray.

Pregnancy may or may not affect your hair. Some women have magnificent curly hair. This may be a blessing, depending upon current hair-styles. Nevertheless, pregnancy sometimes straightens the curl, temporarily or permanently, and there is nothing you can do about it. Further, your hair may become dryer, requiring you to change your shampooing habits. Finally, sometimes after you deliver—usually during the second to fourth month postpartum—you may notice a sudden loss of scalp hair. This hair regrows, and the scalp hair density begins to appear normal in about six months, though for some women regrowth may take much longer. *In very rare cases,* it will not regrow at all and your hair will remain permanently somewhat thinner. Remembering this when you go home after delivery, you should avoid any trauma to your hair for the first six months. Thus, postpone, if you can, the use of rollers, pin curls, permanent-wave solutions, ratting, straightening, and other abusive hair treatment. You should use a natural-bristle hairbrush, but keep vigorous hair-brushing to a minimum. Shampoo as often as necessary.

Your Skin

Your skin undergoes many changes during pregnancy. For one, it is stretched like a drumhead by growing breasts, a growing abdomen, body weight gain, and retained fluid. For another, it is subject to the influence of the hormones produced and secreted throughout pregnancy. With these two powerful inside factors—stretch and hormones—aided and abetted by the inroads of the atmosphere and any harsh beauty products, your skin is likely to feel like the cover of a used weather balloon—and it may not look much better to you. On the other hand, there are women who have had skin problems all their lives who find, to their great joy, that everything on their surface clears up magically during pregnancy: their skin becomes shimmering, healthy, and more attractive than it has ever been. This "bloom of pregnancy" is wonderful to behold. Enjoy!

Acne
The hormone changes that we mentioned may have adverse effects on the skin in early pregnancy and thus bring about changes on the face and neck that resemble acne. These lesions generally clear up as time goes on and should be managed by keeping your skin very clean and using a simple soap and little makeup. Medications are available for severe acne but are rarely needed for pregnancy-induced episodes.

Chloasma
Some women experience chloasma, a mottled darkening of the facial skin that usually becomes heaviest on the forehead, the bridge of the nose, and the cheeks below the eyes. This darkness usually disappears some-

time after delivery. Similar skin darkening may occur around the nipples and certain other body areas but, again, lightens after delivery. Avoid direct sunlight if you have this condition or you may become permanently tanned in those areas. Sunlight exposure is not good for you anyway.

Striae
One of the most distressing of the skin changes that may appear is a series of reddish lines on the abdomen, flanks, and breasts. These striae are more likely to occur in women with delicate skin. They represent the separation of deeper layers of the skin itself, allowing the reddish blood vessels and tissue underneath to show through. Some months after delivery, the redness vanishes and the lines become silvery white and much less noticeable. However, they are not likely to ever completely disappear. Little can be done to prevent striae from appearing, but it may help to do the following:

- •Wear garments that provide good support for the breasts and the abdomen during pregnancy.

- •Maintain a moderate weight gain.

- •Massage your breasts and abdomen at least once daily with a good, penetrating skin cream.

Red Dots
Very often, little red dots, caused by heavily functioning pituitary hormones, appear on the neck and arms in midpregnancy and increase in number and size gradually as time goes on. Not very noticeable—except to the bearer—they are harmless and disappear sometime after your pregnancy is over.

A word of caution here, though. Melanomas complicate 1–2 per 1,000 pregnancies and comprise 8 percent of all malignancies generated during pregnancy. This is a rapidly growing problem because of the increasing danger of sun exposure in a thinning atmosphere and the increased use of tanning beds. The little red dots described above are homogeneous in color and regular in outline. Any irregularly shaped, irregularly pigmented skin growth that is regularly extending its size, whether it preceded your pregnancy or was acquired while pregnant, needs professional evaluation. Don't pass it off.

Superficial Veins
All the superficial veins under your skin, under the influence of certain hormones, dilate while you are pregnant. These dilated vessels produce a

variety of noticeable effects. The larger veins of your arms and hands, legs and feet become distended. Those of the lower extremities tend to stand out even more because of the increasing pressure of your growing pregnancy. Further, it is not unusual to notice a mottling effect on your lower extremities and in the palms of the hands. There is nothing abnormal whatsoever about these changes, and they are only temporary. The treatment of abnormal varicose veins is discussed later on.

Rashes

There are several skin rashes that may bother you during pregnancy:

- Iron supplements may produce a small pinpoint rash over your chest, abdomen, and back. Stop your vitamin-mineral supplement for a week—if your doctor agrees—and it will be gone if it is iron-induced. Then you and your doctor must seek a different iron preparation.

- You may have an itchy sensation all over, generally with no visible rash at all. This little teaser is known as pruritis of pregnancy. No one knows the cause, but nothing serious comes of it—unless your fingernails are too sharp. Try bathing daily in lukewarm water to which you have added a moisturizing lotion. After toweling, apply a lanolin cream, and do so again at bedtime. If your itch seems unbearable, your doctor may prescribe a cortisone-based cream.

- You may have herpes of pregnancy. This skin disorder of unknown cause is totally related to pregnancy and is in no way related to the herpes class of diseases. It usually begins toward midpregnancy, but it may start after delivery. You are covered with an itchy eruption, mainly on your arms, abdomen, upper chest, back, and thighs. (What's left?) This particular rash must be diagnosed and treated by your doctor or by a dermatologist. Rarely, this skin disorder may endanger pregnancy, but, again, it is not related to any dangerous herpes virus.

- You may have allergic rashes as a reaction to anything during pregnancy, just as at any other time. Thus, strawberries, tomatoes, nylon, pollen, jewelry, makeup—anything can give you "contact dermatitis." Watch what you put on your skin and what you eat to nourish it.

Tanning

Although there are no known pregnancy-related risks, as I said earlier, tanning is harmful to you. No matter what you read or are told, the ultraviolet rays that tan you—no matter how they are produced—also increase your risk of future skin cancer and of having damaged and not-too-pretty skin as you get older. Tanning is a protective maneuver devised by your skin in which deep-lying, melanin-containing skin cells migrate to the skin surface to screen out damaging ultra-violet rays. Voilà—you tan. Unfortunately, the constant irritation of melanin skin cells is what leads to melanosarcomas—very dangerous malignant growths. And even if you don't develop cancer, your skin still sustains grievous photodamage over time. Looking into the weathered face of a fine old mariner, you can see what your skin future holds—at the least. Sun-worshiping should be abandoned.

Exercise

We need to remember that we are descended from wandering hunters. As such, our forebears exercised (wandered and hunted) or starved! Incidentally, labor and delivery in those remote times was supposedly a snap. The anecdotes relate that women had their babies while in the foraging fields and continued on with their work—after disposing of the placenta! The journals of Lewis and Clark, for example, describe a Shoshone woman, named Sacajawea, who helped transport the expedition's baggage across the Bitterroot River while she was in active labor. The truth was that she labored long and hard afterwards without progress until she received a labor-stimulating tea made from ground rattles of the rattlesnake tail. Let's not kid ourselves. Labor and delivery in the good old days was not so very good.

Civilization, however, with all its "advantages," has markedly reduced our wandering and hunting to the point that less than 20 percent of us engage in activity sufficient to promote acceptable cardiovascular fitness. Partly because of our inactivity, we have further added a massive new problem—obesity. Fat has become a major health problem in the United States. Recognizing these fat and sedentary facts, health professionals have properly pushed us into a "fitness frenzy." Jogging, walking, swimming, aerobics of all kinds, pumping iron, all manner of mechanical go-nowhere, climb-nowhere, ride-nowhere, row-nowhere devices—all of these things and more have replaced hunting and foraging and carrying baggage across the Bitterroot River. Pregnant women, now concerned about these problems, are therefore increasingly asking their doctors for advice about starting or continuing exercise while they are pregnant. So—let's get to it.

During pregnancy important physiological changes that affect your exercise patterns take place in your body:

•Your connective tissue (which holds together your bones, muscles, joints, and organs) becomes softer, and thus joints and tissues become more susceptible to injury.

•Your blood volume increases dramatically. During exercise, while the blood supply to your brain and heart remains constant, it is diverted away from major abdominal organs, including your uterus, and therefore your fetus. This can be particularly dangerous if anemia (low red blood cell count) is also present.

•Respiratory ventilation decreases and pulmonary reserve cannot always compensate for oxygen intake and carbon dioxide excretion during exercise. Thus, the risk of blood and tissue lactic acid accumulation (acidosis) increases.

•Nutritionally, pregnant women need 300 extra calories a day, and very active women need much more. These needs must be met—particularly if you are on an exercise program—to avoid weight loss and acidosis from lactic acid accumulation.

•The pregnant woman is much more likely to suffer dehydration and heat loss, owing to a number of changes, not the least of which is increased body surface. These two conditions can very quickly and very seriously alter fetal well-being.

•Blood sugar levels can fall very rapidly during pregnancy, and at a much greater rate while exercising strenuously.

•Fetal activity—which includes changes in fetal heart and respiratory rates, fetal temperature, and fetal movements—reflects maternal exercise activity.

•Your physical center of gravity changes as your baby and uterus grow, significantly affecting your balance.

•There will be—and you should anticipate—a progressive decline in performance as pregnancy advances. This decrease may be as little as 10 percent in the early days and mount to 50 percent at the end.

Based on this information and other considerations, the following recommendations have been formulated for exercise during pregnancy by the American College of Obstetricians and Gynecologists; your doctor can get a copy of them for you. They are pretty stout recommendations, but we'll soften them a bit at the end.

1. Maternal heart rate should not exceed 140 beats per minute.

2. Strenuous activities should not exceed 15 minutes in duration.

3. No exercise should be performed on one's back after the fourth month of gestation is completed. (Remember prone-pressure disorder?)

4. Exercises, such as weight-lifting, that employ the Valsalva maneuver (increasing intra-chest pressure by forced exhalation) should be avoided.

5. Caloric intake should be adequate to meet the extra energy needs of not only the pregnancy but also the exercise.

6. Maternal core temperature should not exceed 38°C (100.4°F).

7. Regular exercise (at least three times per week) is preferable to intermittent activity. Competitive activities are discouraged.

8. Vigorous exercise should not be performed in hot, humid weather or during fever.

9. Ballistic movements (jerky, bouncy motions) should be avoided. Exercise should not be done on a wooden floor or a tightly carpeted surface to reduce shock.

10. Deep flexion or extension of joints should be avoided because of connective tissue softening. Activities that require jumping, jarring motions or rapid changes in direction should be avoided because of joint instability.

11. Vigorous exercise should be preceded by a five-minute period of muscle warm-up. This can be established by slow walking or stationary cycling with low resistance.

12. Because connective tissue softening increases the risk of joint injury, vigorous exercise should be followed by a period of gradually declining activity that includes gentle stationary stretching. Stretches should not be taken to the point of maximum resistance.

13. Heart rate should be measured at times of peak activity. Target heart rates and limits established in consultation with a physician should not be exceeded.

14. Care should be taken to rise gradually from the floor to avoid orthostatic hypotension, a sudden drop in blood pressure that often occurs when one assumes an erect posture too quickly. Some form of activity involving the legs should be continued for a brief period.

15. Liquids should be taken liberally before and after exercise to prevent dehydration. If necessary, activity should be interrupted to replenish fluids.

16. Women who have led sedentary lifestyles should begin with physical activity of a very low intensity and advance activity levels very gradually.

17. Activity should be stopped and the physician consulted if any unusual symptoms appear.

This list contains some very valuable but rigid rules for your exercise life. In general, the following exercise guidelines hold up as far as appropriateness and safety are concerned—and they are a little softer.

- Mild to moderate exercise does not have to be omitted in normal pregnancy.

- Overheating, for reasons already made clear, must be avoided.

- Specific exercises within reason need not be avoided.

- Jogging, when it is reasonable and gradually reduced as time goes on, is acceptable.

- Aerobic exercise, scientifically programmed, on soft surfaces, avoiding hyperextension of the back and doing slow warm-ups and cooldowns, is fine. Many aerobic pregnancy videotapes are available today—so many that your physician would have to judge the safety of any particular one for you.

- Bicycling is preferable on a stationary mount indoors. If outdoors and moving, temperature and your skill level are important limitations.

- Swimming is probably the best aerobic exercise for pregnant women. Avoid water that is too hot, too cold, or unclean.

If you are involved in weight-lifting, you may continue, cautiously, using light weights only. Avoid free weights and observe proper breathing techniques when lifting and returning fixed weights.

Relative Contraindications to Exercise During Pregnancy

Your physician will need to evaluate you individually with respect to an exercise program. The following conditions may require you to avoid vigorous physical activity during pregnancy:

•hypertension

•anemia or other blood disorders

•thyroid disease

•cardiac arrhythmia or palpitations

•history of precipitous labor

•history of intrauterine growth retardation (IUGR)

•history of bleeding during present pregnancy

•breech presentation in the last trimester

•excessive obesity or extreme underweight

•history of an extremely sedentary lifestyle

Absolute Contraindications to Exercise During Pregnancy

The following conditions are considered absolute contraindications to vigorous exercise during pregnancy:

•history of three or more miscarriages

•ruptured membranes

•history of premature labor

•diagnosed multiple gestation

•incompetent cervix

•bleeding or a diagnosis of placenta previa (the placenta below baby and over the cervix)

•diagnosed cardiac disease

You must be aware, of course, that certain complications arising during pregnancy may make vigorous activity inadvisable even if you were previously able to exercise without restrictions.

The Sporting Life

Certain sports carry a risk of injury that is substantially greater because, as you know, your joints are now more loosely put together and easier to strain, your footing and balance are not secure, and your body tends to heat up and lose fluids more rapidly. Besides the well-known risk of over-heating, some games involve a risky level of body contact. For these reasons, some restrictions are advisable. Here are considerations for specific sports:

- **Hunting and fishing.** These sports are generally fairly benign. However, if you're going fishing, the wind is up, and your companion is an idiot turned loose with a 100-horsepower motor on a 12-foot canoe, or you are hunting and your shotgun has the recoil factor of a sidewinder missile, take care! Make sure that you are following your general exercise guidelines rather than Rambo's.

- **Tennis, golf, and bowling.** No unusual problems. Remember, though, that your fingers may swell in late pregnancy and they can get stuck in your bowling ball. Watch out for overheating in golf and tennis. The time will come in golf when your swing can't get by your baby.

- **Water sports.** Swimming is the best aerobic activity for a pregnant woman. The water must be neither too hot nor too cold, and it must be clean. Snorkeling at surface levels is fine, but scuba diving represents a great danger to your babe. Water skiing should be avoided because the accidental rush of water into the vagina upon a fall could be disastrous. Incidentally, the same is true of water slides.

- **Snow sports.** Skiing poses certain real hazards other than just injury. Most often you arrive at the high altitudes of ski resorts by plane and thus are suddenly dumped into a low-oxygen atmosphere. This is hard on you, and even more so on your baby. You should avoid any real physical activity for 24 or preferably 48 hours while your system adjusts. Otherwise, your baby may have a real oxygen deficit. If, of course, you already live as high above sea level as your ski resort, then you need not restrict yourself. Cross-country skiing is safer for you both than downhill (Alpine) skiing, but if you are an accomplished skier, green square or a modest blue bullet are probably safe enough. Black diamonds, deep powder, and snowboarding should wait until next winter. Ice skating and snowmobiles should also be avoided.

- **Softball.** This sport is somewhat dangerous in terms of not only potential injury but also fluid loss and overheating. It is better to be team manager.

- **Competitive sports.** Sports involving regular training and stressful exercises are out. There is real danger to the pregnancy.

Professional athletes are a special case; they have a difficult task in reconciling their professional goals with the experiences of childbirth, breast-feeding, and caring for their young. Despite all this, pregnancy can sometimes be managed during a competing season with certain caveats:

Preconceptional counseling is necessary.

Adequate nutrition, vitamins, and minerals must be provided.

The risk of orthopedic injuries must be understood—along with the very real potential for permanent ligament and joint damage.

Overheating and dehydration must be avoided—particularly in early pregnancy.

Every athlete should remember that sports involving sudden changes in height and/or sudden tension on the body (such as free flying, skydiving, and scuba and tower diving) can have serious fetal effects.

Remember also that the following warning signs and symptoms need to be heeded:

• absent or declining fetal activity

• difficulty in walking or moving about, back pain, or any other unusual pain

• dizziness, falling out, a very rapid pulse or palpitations

• pubic bone discomfort or pain (This bony juncture at the very bottom of your abdomen can actually separate in pregnancy.)

• vaginal bleeding or watery discharge

• uterine cramps

The benefits of regular sporting activity outweigh many of the risks—pregnant or not. Remember, though, that risks do exist and that you and/or your baby may be hurt in almost any physical activity. Sport with care, sport!

The American College of Obstetricians and Gynecologists, as well as other sources, can supply your doctor with printed sport and exercise information for you.

Working

Not too long ago, being pregnant and gainfully employed outside the home presented no problem at all. As soon as pregnancy declared itself,

the bearer was fired, perhaps to be rehired sometime in the future—perhaps not. This was the archaic state of affairs until quite recently. As
more and more women entered the workforce, business attitudes began
to change, mainly as a result of some women having the nerve to challenge their employer's discriminatory practices in court. There is still a
long way to go, but we are moving along rapidly. Big and small busi-
nesses have become aware that to dismiss pregnant women from their
service out of hand is to squander immense talent and enrichment of
their ranks. Moreover, government intervention has forced laggard
employers into the modern world.

Women began entering the workforce during World War II and have
gradually increased their presence ever since. They continue to work now
for a number of reasons: the need for second-salary support in modern
households; their increasing desire to follow career goals; and the decision to delay achieving their reproductive goals.

Pregnancy often complicates and at least temporarily alters these reasons for working. A recent national study revealed that:

- Slightly over 60 percent of American mothers aged 15 to 44
  worked for pay six months or so before their latest delivery. Of
  these, 46.1 percent worked full-time, and 14 percent part-time.

- Nearly 80 percent of women worked during their third trimester,
  and more than 50 percent worked up to less than one month before
  delivery.

Here are some other interesting points:

- The U.S. Department of Labor reports that 44 percent of the
  pregnant workforce is employed in technical, sales, and
  administrative occupations; 26.2 percent in managerial and
  professional jobs; 17.7 percent in service; 8.5 percent as operators,
  fabricators, and laborers; 2.2 percent in craft, repair, and precision
  positions; and 1.1 percent in farming, forestry, and fishing.

- Many studies have been done on the effect of various jobs on
  pregnancy. They can be summarized by saying that most pregnant
  working women do very well except in work that demands heavy
  lifting, standing for long periods, high degrees of stress, or
  exposure to certain toxins.

- Observers have noted the "healthy worker effect": pregnant
  workers in an appropriate job environment appear to have better
  outcomes than does the general unemployed pregnant population.

•The Occupational Safety and Health Administration, the Women's Defense and Legal Fund, and a host of federal and state legislation have cleared the way for pregnant women to work safely and, if healthy and not in a dangerous environment, to continue to work while pregnant, to have up to 12 weeks of unpaid leave, and to have job security when they return. Even with these improvements, however, our country lags far behind most developed nations in its family and work policies.

To get down to basics, certain factors must be considered when making decisions about your work and your pregnancy.

First, your health.

There are certain obstetrical complications that warrant restrictions in how long you work. They include:

•previous delivery of two premature infants, whether due to a weakened cervix, congenital deformities of the uterus, or other unknown causes

•significant heart disease

•significant high blood pressure

•severe diabetes

•severe anemia or other important blood disorders

•systemic diseases such as kidney disorders, convulsive states, and crippling orthopedic limitations

Many of these limitations are relative; how they affect your job depends upon their seriousness and the type of work you perform. Your physician can help you with these decisions.

There are also, of course, a number of strictly obstetrical complications that can force you either to terminate your work or to make modifications. These include:

•vaginal bleeding

•ruptured membranes

•hypertension of pregnancy

•abnormal placental location

•multiple infants

These events, too, may be subject to some modification by multiple conditioning factors. Again, your physician is your source of help here. Moreover, other obstetrical problems not mentioned here may require you to stay home.

The Type of Work You Do

Certain work environments may pose specific hazards to pregnancy. These include—but are not limited to—the following:

- •Work that may expose you to ionizing radiation (X-rays). Thus, certain hospital, clinic, and dental offices are off-limits unless absolute protection is provided for you.

- •Work that exposes you to hazardous and toxic materials, including lead, ethylene oxide, propane, and certain anesthetic gases.

- •Work in environments, such as laboratories, dialysis units, certain hospital areas, pet shops, and school classrooms, that exposes you to dangerous bacteria, certain antineoplastic drugs, and organic solvents.

- •Work that requires putting in long hours under high stress.

- •Excessive physical work, long hours of standing, work requiring physical dexterity and motion.

Numerous flawed news reports have frightened women by suggesting that computers, microwave ovens, and even electric blankets may be harmful to the developing fetus. However, there is no firm evidence that any of this is factual.

Company Policy

As mentioned earlier, company policies toward pregnant employees have changed dramatically in the last few years. Most organizations consider their employees to be assets on their balance sheets and treat them accordingly. *Working Mother,* a magazine devoted to the cares, concerns, and nurturing of working mothers, publishes an annual list of the 100 best American companies with respect to how they address the concerns of these employees. It is a revelation to read about such companies and the revolution they have produced. From Allstate to Xerox, they have introduced family leaves with job-back security, flexibility, home working, child care, advancement opportunity—you name it, they've done it. You will benefit from reading this surprising and exciting information. (Available at newsstands, *Working Mother* is published by MacDonald Communications, 135 W. 50th St., New York, N.Y. 10020.)

Suffice to say that company policy now rarely prevents pregnant women from working as long as they wish or can. The only limitations are those related to hazardous occupations. After all, business must protect itself as well as its workers.

Finally, leaves of absence have become more readily obtainable for short-term problems such as severe early nausea and vomiting or for blood pressure control later on.

Return to Work

This may be your salvation. It is very good to get out into the real world again—particularly if your work environment is supportive and child care arrangements are easily made. Customarily, women have returned to work, after either a normal delivery or a cesarean section, in six weeks—unless their postpartum course has been complicated. At present, however, these limitations have become more flexible; depending on the type of work you do, your health, your wishes, and your physician's blessing, you may return to your job earlier. Or later!

More Pregnant Pauses

•Many pregnant women do, in fact, crave ice cream. Häagen-Dazs is a very popular dessert in America. The same is true in Japan. But whereas our favorites are vanilla and chocolate, the flavors green tea, sesame, and wasabi take the cake there—or go with the cake!

•There are many ancient remedies for morning sickness. Some of them would sicken you. I can remember a treatment that involved a red-hot poker, a sliver of ice, and a piece of meat. The poor vomiting mother, lying in bed with her abdomen screened, would see the approaching doctor wielding the red-hot poker, which, he explained, he was about to lay upon her abdomen to end her nausea. Instead, he laid the ice on her abdomen and the poker on the bit of meat! That was early smoking, sizzling shock therapy. If the poor mother didn't miscarry, she certainly never complained about vomiting again.

  Ancient Chinese therapy for nausea involved acupressure on the Neiguan point inside the wrist. Recently, wristbands that apply pressure on this area were tested against bands that do not. The result? Two-thirds of the women were helped by the real bands, while just one-third of the controls described having only some relief. Apparently, you can't beat the band.

•Many mothers who are heavy smokers and can't seem to quit, even knowing the risks to their babies, will manage to do so after watching their first ultrasound procedure. Something about the little child's heartbeat or body movements turns the mother on and nicotine off.

•More than half of all pregnant women suffer from morning sickness during the first few months, and half of those feel its effects all day. About one in ten have morning sickness before they miss a period, and women who plan their pregnancies are more likely to be afflicted. Women whose sisters were nauseated are also more likely to be nauseated themselves. There appears to be no relationship between morning sickness and age, race, weight, type of work, marital status, or previous pregnancies. Women who smoke are less likely to be nauseated than those who don't. That is an observation, not an encouragement. Don't ever smoke— pregnant or not.

•Men can have early nausea and vomiting alongside their mates. They also have been observed to suffer from pregnancy pica: the desire—even need—to ingest nonfood substances.

•You can sleep on a waterbed. That's what your babe is sleeping in.

•Having problems at work with dangerous areas, toxins, or smoke? Help is available from:
  The National Institute for Occupational Safety and Health, 4676
    Columbia Pkwy., Cincinnati, OH 45226 (800–356–4674).
  U.S. Department of Labor, Women's Bureau Clearinghouse
    (800–827–5335). Get a copy of the bureau's brochure
    "Pregnancy Discrimination—Know Your Rights."

Diary

My Second Month

Problems_____

_____

Illness_____

_____

Medications_____

_____

Spotting_____

_____

Persistent nausea, etc._____

_____

Travel_____

_____

Ultrasound—why?_____

_____

What's going on in the world?_____

_____

_____

_____

What's going on in my life?_____

_____

_____

_____

My thoughts and feelings_____

_____

_____

_____

Doctor's appointment_____

Questions to ask_____

_____

_____

_____

_____

_____

_____

_____

_____

_____

_____

_____

_____

_____

_____

_____

_____

_____

_____

_____

_____

_____

_____

_____

_____

_____

_____

Three

My Third Lunar Month

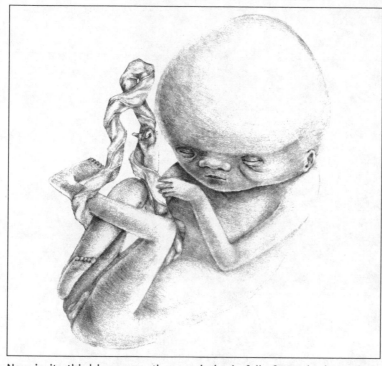

Now in its third lunar month, your baby is fully formed, about three inches long, and as big as a large rosebud. Its heart is now a formed and beating structure. Although this fetus is moving about regularly, such activity is too slight for you to feel. Your uterus—its home—is as big as a large orange.

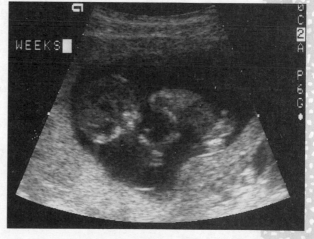

The ultrasound clearly reveals the baby's whole body, and its movements, as well as the beating heart, can be seen. It is not too early to establish certain normal and reassuring structural landmarks.

Now, nearing the point of missing your third period and thus entering the third lunar month of your pregnancy, you are about to pass another physiological landmark. Several changes take place. One of them concerns the hormone progesterone, which, as you know, is vitally important to the maintenance of pregnancy. Until now, this hormone has been secreted almost entirely by a corpus luteum cyst on the ovary from whence ovulation took place, but hereafter it will be secreted by the placenta (afterbirth), while the corpus luteum slowly withers away. This transference of hormone manufacture does not always progress smoothly. It is at this time in pregnancy, therefore, that one type of spontaneous abortion may take place.

Before opening a full-scale discussion of spontaneous abortion, I want to detail a very new approach to dating early pregnancy changes that fits more accurately the events that lead to pregnancy loss. Instead of dividing pregnancy into three trimesters, the newer approach, based upon the work of Steven R. Goldstein, M.D., logically follows the upcoming infant's early growth pattern. In the beginning, each pregnancy consists of a small "gestational sac" embedded within the uterine lining. Shortly thereafter, an ultrasound can pick up a yolk sac with a little embryo strip attached to its surface. All this is less than three millimeters in size. Soon an embryo can be seen that measures up to five millimeters, and next, five to ten millimeters, and finally, up to ten millimeters or more. We are now approaching seventy days since the last menstrual period (LMP), and a recognizable fetus is now present. Thus, we have left the embryo period and entered the fetal period.

Here is the importance of approaching pregnancy development this way:

Pregnancy Stage	Chance of Pregnancy Loss
Gestational sac	11.5%
Yolk sac	8.8
Embryo to 5 mm.	7.1
Embryo 5–10 mm.	3.3
Embryo 10 mm. or greater	0.5

Although these are the very accurate determinations of the actual times when fetal demise may have occurred, they are not necessarily the times when the pregnancy physically leaves the uterus in the form of a miscarriage. That often happens weeks later. But based upon these observations, embryo or fetal death can be determined early on. Of equal importance, as these figures reveal, once the pregnancy reaches the fetal stage with a beating heart (70 days from the LMP), subsequent miscarriage is very unlikely. These exquisite ultrasound determinations, often combined with beta HCG, can faultlessly monitor a pregnancy as it progresses, eliminate or confirm an ectopic pregnancy almost without fail, and date a pregnancy to within three days—a feat that can save a ton of problems further down the road.

Spontaneous Abortion

Strictly speaking, *abortion* is a medical term that means the loss of a pregnancy before the fetus can survive—generally considered to be 20 weeks or under 500 grams in weight (just over one pound). With modern neonatal intensive care, some of these "abortions" are living and possibly well today. The popular term for an abortion is *miscarriage*—but they are one and the same.

The most usual time for a miscarriage is around the twelfth week, but we have seen that that may not be the time of embryonic or fetal demise. Here are some abortion terms that may interest you.

- •**Complete.** The pregnancy has completely expelled itself—fetus or embryo plus placenta—from the uterus.

- •**Incomplete.** This common event involves the expulsion of only parts of the pregnancy. The cervix is open, there is bleeding and cramping, but some elements of the pregnancy remain in the uterus.

- •**Missed.** The fetus or embryo is no longer living, but it remains within the uterus. Four weeks after death is the diagnostic time limit, but that figure varies greatly. Today such prolonged retentions—if diagnosed—are not allowed to continue.

Here are some statistics about spontaneous abortions that you may wish to know.

- •The estimates of how frequently spontaneous abortions occur vary considerably—anywhere from 12 to 30 percent. As we become able to diagnose pregnancies earlier and with greater certainty, the rate of proven early loss increases. Moreover, as more and more pregnancies are attempted by older women and by those who run a high risk of infertility, the rate of spontaneous abortion is bound to increase.

•After one or more spontaneous abortions, the chance of one recurrence is somewhat greater.

•Four percent of the population of women have sustained two spontaneous abortions and 3 percent have experienced three.

•The frequency of spontaneous abortion in 20-year-old women is around 12 percent. This rate doubles for women 40 and over.

•Because of our advancing knowledge, our increased diagnostic capabilities, and the changes in the pregnant population, these statistics change as we write. It is worth remembering, as we will see in a moment, that most abortions are the result of nature's close scanning for imperfect embryos.

What Brings About Spontaneous Abortions?

We cannot yet determine the cause of each spontaneous abortion as it physically takes place. Over the long run, however, the sum of all causes is pretty clearly established.

•**Genetics.** As we have already seen, nature scans each pregnancy for life-incompatible genetic errors and promptly aborts almost all of them—sometimes before women realize that they are pregnant. At other times, the pregnancy may not succumb until the late embryo stage, and as we have seen, the physical event of abortion may not happen until even later. Rarely, genetic defects that are not life-threatening—at least within the uterine environment—escape nature's scythe. Thus, we have Down's syndrome and certain other survivable genetic problems to deal with at full term. However, at least 97 percent of all genetic abnormalities are aborted by natural forces, and these account for about 50 percent of all spontaneous abortions. Genetic counseling and study should be undertaken once this diagnosis is established.

•**Anatomical problems.** Such problems include malformations of the uterus caused by tumors (fibroids being a perfect example), congenital mishaps (a double uterus, for instance), and incompetence of the cervix (see page 233). Corrective surgery for such problems often makes the uterus a friendly pregnancy environment.

•**Glandular disorders.** You are already aware of progesterone's role in spontaneous abortion, but other glandular substances may be involved. Disorders in the thyroid, adrenal, or pituitary gland may all influence pregnancy health very significantly. Proper studies to identify and neutralize the culprit reduce abortion risks.

•**Infections.** A number of infections are known to lead to a poor pregnancy outcome. Toxoplasmosis, mycoplasmosis, chlamydia, and group B beta hemolytic streptococcus are maternal infections that can lead to abortion. Toxoplasmosis is transmitted by animals—usually cats—while the others are transmitted by the human animal. Appropriate antibiotic therapy is the required treatment.

•**Self-abuse.** Both nicotine and alcohol abuse contribute to spontaneous abortions.

•**Toxins.** Certain work and environmental toxins (see chapter 2) can contribute to this problem.

•**Immunological problems.** About 15 percent of *recurrent* spontaneous abortions may be related to the complex area of autoimmune disorders. Antinuclear antibodies, lupus anticoagulant, anticardiolipin antibodies, or others may be involved in producing clots under the placenta, resulting in fetal death. Cortisone, heparin, and aspirin in various combinations are being used at present in study programs to try to avert clotting. This work is exceedingly complicated—to diagnose, to treat, and to talk about. To date, the results of these pharmaceutical interventions are difficult to assess but appear to offer some help.

•**Maternal age and illnesses.** We have already seen that age is an abortion factor. So also are certain maternal illnesses such as diabetes, liver, kidney, and heart disease, and the glandular problems noted earlier.

You can now appreciate what a complex problem we have to deal with here. Nevertheless, there are four facts you should remember:

1. Most abortions are nature's preventive scanning at work.

2. *Recurrent* abortions are an uncommon obstetrical condition.

3. Significant help is available for women prone to recurrent abortions.

4. Once 70 days from your last period elapse and a beating heart is visible by ultrasound, the spontaneous abortion rate is almost zero.

There are two other categories of abortion. A *therapeutic* abortion is indicated when the mother has a life-threatening disorder that will not allow her to carry a baby to term and live. An *elective* abortion is a procedure chosen when the mother, for her own reasons, feels she cannot cope with a pregnancy.

Symptoms of a Spontaneous Abortion

The symptoms of impending abortion are vaginal bleeding and menstrual-like cramping—although you may experience both of these symptoms to a noticeable degree without an abortion being imminent, or even in the cards. But it is very important that you tell your doctor about any such events and that he or she be involved in your care. Again, some early vaginal bleeding and some uterine cramping are not uncommon and may truly mean nothing, but you need to let your doctor know and you need to avoid any unnecessary activity until a diagnosis is established.

Spontaneous Abortion Treatment

- A *complete* abortion requires no treatment at all.

- An *incomplete* abortion usually requires an outpatient D&C (dilation of the cervix and curettage [scraping] of the uterine lining). Often the cervix is already dilated or open, so only a curettage is necessary. Also, sometimes instead of curetting the uterus, a suction device is inserted into the uterine cavity and the remaining tissue is sucked away. Rarely, the patient suffers enough blood loss that hospital admission is necessary. Since the demise of criminal abortions, infection is rarely present.

- A *missed* abortion needs to be evacuated from the uterus either by a D&C or by the suctioning technique. Delay is not wise. Established absence of cardiac activity along with a declining beta HCG level makes the diagnosis firm.

Rhogam—the Rh vaccine—must be given to all Rh-negative mothers who abort and to all mothers of unknown Rh type—a rare unknown nowadays.

Medical Abortions

This abortion overview would not be complete without a discussion of the drug techniques used to procure an abortion—usually with no surgical intervention. A great public outcry followed the news that European

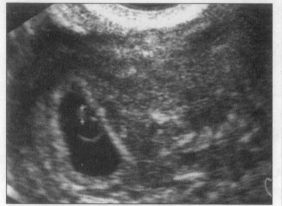

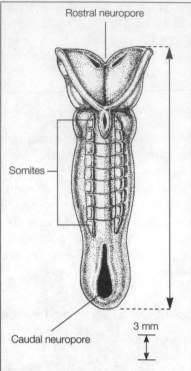

The ultrasound above reveals a pregnancy of 31 days duration (45 days from the LMP—Last Menstrual Period). The chorionic villi have embedded into the uterus and a placenta will soon be forming. An embryo can be seen between the two cross marks; to the right is a schematic drawing of that three-millimeter embryo. With high resolution ultrasound, a beating heart tube can be seen! *(Courtesy of* Contemporary OB/GYN *and Steven R. Goldstein, M.D.)*

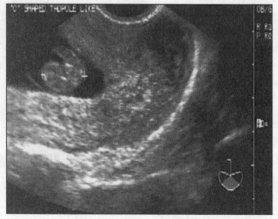

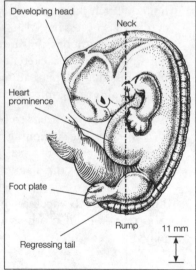

Above is an ultrasound taken 55 days after the LMP (41 days actual pregnancy duration). The embryo measures 11 millimeters from crown to rump, and has a head, a tail, and a beating heart. On the right, again, is a schematic drawing. *(Courtesy of* Contemporary OB/GYN *and Steven R. Goldstein, M.D.)*

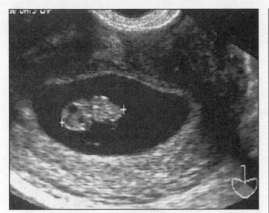

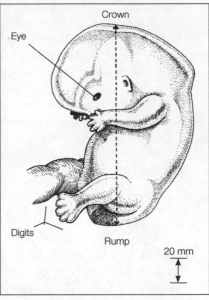

This ultrasound was taken 60 days (5 weeks) after the LMP (46 days of pregnancy). The crown rump (between the cross marks) measures 20 millimeters, the tail is gone, and eyes and digits appear as can be seen on the drawing at the right. The umbilical cord is clearly visible. *(Courtesy of* Contemporary OB/GYN *and Steven R. Goldstein, M.D.)*

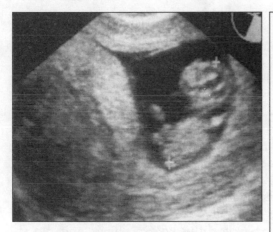

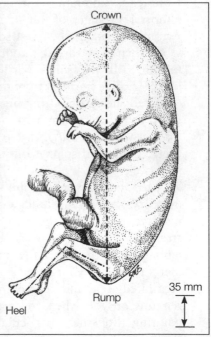

An ultrasound taken at day 70 from the LMP (56 days pregnant). We are no longer dealing with an embryo but a true fetus—a miniature baby as the drawing at the right shows. Arriving at this point with a proper crown-rump length (about 35 millimeters), a beating heart, and no visible significant deformities, this pregnancy will very, very rarely miscarry. *(Courtesy of* Contemporary OB/GYN *and Steven R. Goldstein, M.D.)*

pharmaceutical companies had made mifepristone (RU486) generally available. This drug can induce an abortion in most instances. Its potential introduction into the American market is what created the controversy. When, and if, it is released is of little consequence. Already available in this country is methotrexate (see page 18) and a variety of prostaglandin drugs that are widely used to induce labor (see page 254). Combinations of these two agents will reliably produce an abortion for whatever reason the abortion is indicated.

Hobbies

There are over 70 million American hobbyists, and the number continues to grow. With more discretionary time and increasingly automated households, there is more free quality time for everything from collecting spiders to waltzing the Web. Hobbies are an excellent way to relax and a healthy form of self-expression. Few hobbies constitute a real threat to pregnancy, but many chemical compounds find their way into the hobbyist's equipment. Since there are now about two and a half million chemical compounds, with more being added each year, it is important to determine whether any of these may be harmful.

There is truth in the long-standing belief that painting endangers a pregnant woman and her child. Certain pigments in oil paints are derived from lead, cadmium, barium, and other heavy metals. Although there is almost no danger of inhaling these substances while you are painting, you may accidentally ingest some of them from your fingers or they may work their way through your skin. Do not hold brush handles in your mouth. All pigments—particularly lead, which accumulates in the body—can be harmful to both mother and child.

Even though painting may not be your hobby, you may feel called upon to paint a room or some piece of furniture during pregnancy. No matter what, *avoid lead-based paint.* If you paint indoors, use synthetic paint and splat it on in a well-ventilated room. Don't use spray paints.

Most house paints, including latex paints, contain a small amount of mercury to prevent mildew and spoilage. If any of this mercury is ingested or gets to the intestines somehow (via the lungs and bloodstream, for instance), it can be converted to a type of mercury that is damaging to the fetus. Recent studies have shown that there is enough mercury in our paint to cause problems. Be sure that you paint in a well-ventilated area, and keep paint off your body, making certain that none remains on you when you are finished. You might even want to avoid painting altogether—particularly if you splatter-paint like I do!

If your hobbies run to metal sculpture, which carries a risk of noxious gases accumulating, or to the construction of miniature airplanes, autos, trains, space stations, and the like, or to any other conceivable activity involving fumes from glues or sprays, be sure to work in a well-ventilated, constantly air-replacing environment.

Barium, cobalt oxide, and lead are commonly used as glazes in pottery. These agents are toxic, and contact with them, particularly with the lead, should be avoided.

Other materials represent a hazard to you because they can cause lung disorders—for example, the asbestos used in modeling material or the sawdust that results from carpentry work. If your hobby is photography, please stay out of the darkroom and away from its chemicals. They can be inhaled and absorbed transdermally.

New and often exotic hobbies keep emerging—some of them difficult to distinguish from sports or cutting-edge thrills. Sky diving and rock climbing come to mind. Your good common sense will remind you to check out these "hobbies" with medical headquarters.

Clothing

Time was when a pregnant woman outgrew her regular clothes, she retired to her home, out of public view. This is how the word *confinement* came to be related to pregnancy: She literally was confined to her home until the blessed event. There were no special maternity clothes and little or no open discussion about maternity or clothes. What mothers put on their bodies is not known to us. All we know is that they were well covered and lonely as the devil.

Today expectant mothers carry their precious burdens everywhere throughout all of pregnancy. They continue to work, travel, and socialize, and they expect and deserve to be gracefully covered with comfortable garments. My favorite weathercaster for the National Weather Channel is so close to her delivery time that at this moment she has difficulty drawing a deep breath while she follows the weather from Portland to Miami. But she continues to work and to look marvelous in the designer clothes provided for her. I don't know whether she gets to take them home with her or not—but she deserves them.

Anyway, the clothing industry has met the outgoing motherhood challenge with a great variety of good-looking maternity clothes that you should begin to wear as soon as your regular clothes become uncomfortable. This happens at a different time for each expectant mother and each pregnancy, depending on weight and build, number of previous pregnancies, the size of the pregnancy, the number of infants inside you, and what you yourself put into your stomach. When your time for maternity clothes comes, don't fight it. You will be sick and tired of wearing maternity clothes before you are finished, but at least you will be sick and tired in comfort. And you will look good!

Some other points:

•**Swimwear.** Since you may well be swimming sometime, somewhere, while you are pregnant, you will sooner or later put away your bikini and start looking at a new, elegantly designed, one-piece pregnancy suit. These new suits are designed so that you won't look like—or feel like—you just stepped out of an old ad for Model-T Fords. And for anyone who can't give them up, there are actually some good-looking two-piece suits designed so that the top adjusts to the changing conditions beneath it.

•**Giving out.** One gambit when your waist begins to expand is to wear a long, loose-fitting top while continuing to wear old slacks below. Leave the front of your pants open and wear suspenders! Don't laugh. Try it—it works.

•**Poaching.** Try some of his shirts and sweaters to wear around the house on evenings or weekends. They should be loose and comfortable—unless he is a stick!

•It is sometimes necessary—even desirable—to wear a girdle, or even a corset specifically designed for pregnancy. Lightweight supports—particularly with a cotton underpant—such as the Baby Hugger (Trennaventions of Derry, Pennsylvania), often provide comforting uplift as well as pressure relief.

•**Footwear.** Sad to say, your feet will probably increase slightly in size during pregnancy and may stay that way afterward. They may also temporarily increase in size because of local swelling (edema). This second effect is less likely to be a problem if you avoid excessive weight gain, get adequate time to prop your feet up, and avoid constrictive garments or garters below your waist. Wear comfortable and well-fitting shoes. Avoid high heels and pointed toes because they offer a very unstable and often damaging underpinning.

•**Garrotes.** As suggested, never wear round garters to support your hose. Wear either a maternity garter belt or pantyhose designed for pregnant women. If you are troubled with varicose veins during your pregnancy, fairly attractive support hose and support pantyhose can be purchased. Pregnant or not, you should wear pantyhose with a cotton crotch. Synthetic fibers trap moisture in the vulvo-vaginal area and often result in conditions unpleasant to you. The retained moisture further adds to the potential for vaginal infections and makes treatment more difficult.

•**Bra support.** Do you have to wear a bra during pregnancy? You don't *have* to, but good judgment dictates that you get some support where and when you need it. As we saw in chapter 1, your breasts will be very congested and tender during the first few months at least and will begin to make that watery secretion called colostrum. Remember, colostrum may stain your bra, but if you don't choose to wear one, it will stain the next closest garment. Disposable nursing shields will protect your bra.

A good approach, both now and throughout your pregnancy, is: Don't try and be what you *were*—be what you *are*. Dress to be comfortable as you are, not as you were.

Your Weight

Having lived through the agony and deprivation caused by nausea, it is easy to become obsessed with making up for lost time. Everything edible looks, tastes, smells, even feels good. Your passions may no longer ignite for your old stablemate, or for furs, diamonds, or even Calvin Klein. Instead, you are now turned on by fried chicken, pizza, tacos, creamed potatoes, creamed anything, ice cream, pies, cakes, rolls, cookies, doughnuts, and dough anything. "Food-in-mouth" disease has arrived. Soon, however, the bell on your scales tolls—and it tolls for you. Weight—and its management—is now at your table. Moreover, nutrition is shortly getting ready to sit down. We have a bunch of nutritional problems in our richly endowed America, but we have just two major weight problems, and they are both related to malnutrition.

•Marilyn Monroe (who, if still alive, would now be in her seventies!) wore, and properly filled, a size 12 dress—a dress size that now represents, for many women, a dietary failure. She, however, looked wonderful! Miss America of 1921 weighed 137 pounds and was 5'4" tall, while Miss America of 1987 was 5'8½" tall and 117 pounds! Clearly, thin is in—bringing with it anorexia, bulimia, and malnutrition.

•At the other end of the scales, obesity has become an even more disastrous health problem involving well over one-third of us all. It leads to, among other things, diabetes, heart disease, cancer, and premature death. Next to tobacco, it is the leading "real" cause of death in America, and it is a very bad companion for pregnancy.

Both of these problems are in fact bad companions for pregnancy, and again, both involve malnutrition, our next topic. But right now, dealing with weight and pregnancy fills our plate.

PREGNANCY LOAD FACTORS

Maternal Factors

Growth of breasts, increased uterus and blood volume, water retention, and fat	17 pounds

Fetal Factors

Baby, placenta, and amniotic fluid	10 pounds
Grand total:	27 pounds

There are, of course, a number of variables in these load factors, but they do not—or should not–change the total weight gain by very much. Let's see how two of the maternal factors—fat and fluids—work during pregnancy.

Fat

Our body storage areas contain a set number of fat cells that are like empty balloons when not filled with fat. This set number of fat cells can increase when the storage demand is sufficient. The road to obesity is thus carved—empty fat cells are easier to fill than to build. In our ancient foraging days, the fat storage areas were very important, since we had to gorge and store when food was found. Fat could then be burned later as fuel (and survival) during the lean times. For some basic genetic reason, acquiring, metabolizing, and storing fat is much easier during pregnancy. A modest amount of fat storage is fine, but an excess storage can lead to serious long-term health problems (heart disease, hypertension, stroke, diabetes, cancer) as well as short-term pregnancy problems such as pregnancy diabetes, hypertension, and labor problems. To explore some of the very simplest long-term fat problems, try to imagine what it would be like to carry around 30 pounds of anything each and every day. Besides being carried around, 30 pounds of fat must be fed, housed, heated, cooled, and taken to the bathroom regularly. Think about it. Heavy people just wear out faster.

Fluids

Pregnancy induces certain hormone changes that favor the retention of fluids. Some of it increases the blood volume, but most is retained in tissues outside the bloodstream as edema. Thus, your legs may get puffy, your shoes tight, your fists difficult to make, and your rings difficult to get off and on. Because of gravity, more fluid accumulates in your lower extremities as the day wears on, then is redistributed throughout your upper tissues during the recumbent nighttime—but it doesn't go away.

Only modest swelling should occur. Excessive swelling means something is wrong. Toxemia (hypertension of pregnancy), excess salt intake, anemia, and kidney disturbances are commonly associated with edema and will all be dealt with as we move along. Do not restrict fluid intake to avoid swelling. It does not work and in fact may increase fluid retention. It is, moreover, a very harmful practice.

Now, on to the crux of the matter—your weight gain.

Your Weight and the Body Mass Index

The Body Mass Index (BMI) has become the way to determine what category our weight places us in. Unfortunately, it is not a simple number to produce. It is derived by dividing your weight (in grams) by your height (in meters) squared. Got it?

A BMI between 19.8 and 26 is considered normal. Beneath that, you are underweight, and over it, you're overweight. With a BMI over 29 you are considered obese. Sorry, these are not my rules.

To make it easier for us to work with the BMI, the National Academy of Science has put all this calculus into a chart that shows us how to locate ourselves on the BMI scale. Based on the figure provided for your own BMI, you can determine what weight—and weight gain—is best for you to achieve during your pregnancy.

Maternal BMI Class	Recommended Weight Gain (lbs)	per Month
Underweight (BMI less than 19.8)	28–40	5
Normal weight (BMI 19.8–26)	25–35	4
Overweight (BMI 26.1–29)	15–25	2.6
Obese (BMI over 29)	15	2

These are the guidelines now recommended for single pregnancies. Multiple pregnancies are another matter. For example, twin weight gain should be 35–45 pounds at the rate of 6 pounds each month. Your own

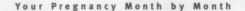

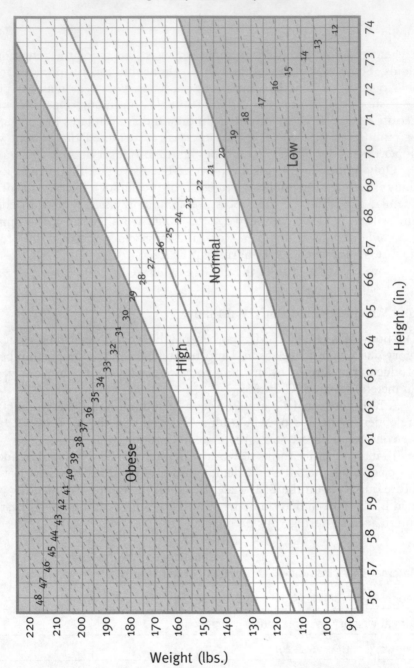

Body mass index (BMI) chart. To find a BMI category (e.g., obese), find the point where the height and weight intersect. To estimate BMI, read the bold number on the dashed line that is closest to this point. *(Institute of Medicine. Subcommittee for a Clinical Application Guide, Committee on Nutritional Status During Pregnancy and Lactation, Food and Nutrition Board, and the National Academy of Sciences. "Nutrition during pregnancy and lactation." Washington, D.C.: National Academy Press, 1992)*

physician should set the goals for your weight gain if you're carrying more than twins.

Finally, here are some uploading weight points:

- Women whose BMI marks them as obese and who gain more than another 25 pounds have numerous increased pregnancy risks— including the increased chance of delivering a macrocosmic (overweight) infant, with all the attendant problems. On the other hand, gaining less than 10 pounds increases the risk of a small infant with other problems.

- No attempt should be made to lose weight during pregnancy. Moreover, if you're losing weight because of nausea and vomiting, your physician needs to know about it at once. Slow weight gain in early pregnancy is not a concern.

- If you have an eating disorder that is not obvious to your doctor, it is very important that you tell him or her about this problem at the earliest possible time.

- There is a positive relationship between maternal weight gain and newborn weight.

- Low prepregnant weight accompanied by inadequate weight gain during pregnancy is a major cause of intrauterine growth retardation (IUGR) (see pages 160–161) and low birth weight.

- Any time weight is lost, it means that the intake of dietary calories is inadequate. Thus, body fat must be burned for fuel. When fat is being broken down, it creates acids—ketones mainly. These ketones must be excreted by the kidneys (ketonuria), but they circulate throughout the body until the kidneys can excrete them. This acid state can have serious fetal effects if it persists for any length of time—an important reason not to try to lose weight at any time during pregnancy.

- Excess weight gained during pregnancy is hard to lose afterward.

Nutrition

Earlier we noted that America has the finest and most varied, complete, and readily available food supply in the world. Almost anyone can find adequate and complete nourishment either through their own means or through private or public sources. Yet we are beset by incredible nutritional problems. Here are some examples:

•The United States now ranks 15th in all the world in infant survival at birth. Although this ranking represents a slight improvement over the past, it is still a dismal figure and hard to believe. One of the major contributing factors to this poor showing is the bad dietary habits of expectant mothers. Without adequate dietary building blocks, it is not possible to develop a healthy baby. These nutritional deficiencies have nothing to do with money—only habits. (Denmark, incidentally, holds the number-one fetal survival spot.)

•Adolescent mothers are more numerous in America than in any other developed country. A growing youngster who becomes pregnant faces many more physiological problems than does her mature, completely developed sister. One of her most serious problems is developing and nourishing another human while her own development is still not complete. The result is many nutritional hazards—even when, rarely, her diet is adequate—and so adolescent mothers lose more children at birth than any other category of pregnant American women.

•Once again, available evidence suggests that the dietary habits of American mothers, both pregnant and not pregnant, are often inadequate and bizarre. The intake of iron, calcium, certain important vitamins, and proteins is well below what it should be. Iron deficiency is very common; many women do not take in enough to meet their own iron needs while pregnant, let alone those of the growing infant. The likelihood of iron-deficiency anemia in both mother and child is very great indeed. The iron supplement provided for pregnant women, even if taken according to instructions, is often inadequate to supply these needs. The same is true of other important vitamins and minerals such as folic acid and calcium.

The National Academy of Science has compiled a list of the basic elements required each day during pregnancy and lactation. This list covers protein, vitamin, and mineral needs but does not include fat and carbohydrate requirements. We'll get to them. Finally, we are provided with the U.S. Department of Agriculture's popular Food Guide Pyramid (see page 79), which spells out for us what our daily bread should be.

Calories and Food

No diet survey would be complete without considering calories—the term given to a unit of energy released by a measured amount of food. A stick of celery offers you almost no calories (you actually burn more

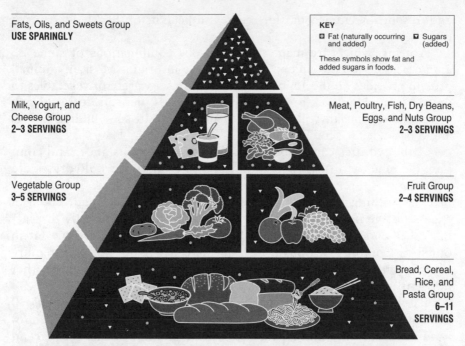

Food Guide Pyramid. *(U.S. Department of Agriculture. "The food guide pyramid." Home and Garden Bulletin no. 252. Washington, D.C.: U.S. Department of Agriculture, Human Nutrition Information Service, 1992)*

calories digesting it than it provides!), while a fudge brownie sundae offers you about 1,130 calories or nearly half your daily caloric needs! In the non-dog-eared pages in most cookbooks you can find the caloric equivalents of most foods. Remember that a gram of fat provides 9 calories while protein and carbohydrates provide 4—less than half that of fat.

The usual daily requirement of 2,000 calories for nonpregnant women increases to about 2,300 during pregnancy. Less (probably a good deal less) than 30 percent of this caloric total should come from **fat,** and that fact generally involves significant revisions in our dietary habits. Moreover, *saturated fats* should be limited at all times because of their potential for producing future cardiac disease. Such fats, as we are now all well aware, come mainly from animals and dairy products but are also abundant in coconut and palm oil. *Polyunsaturated fats,* usually liquid vegetable oils, are considered safer components of your daily fat allowance. However, when these oils are made solid for margarines and pastries by bubbling hydrogen through them, they become trans-fatty acids—almost like saturated fats. *Monounsaturated fats,* which include olive and canola oil, are possibly the safest oils of all. They may even suppress the formation of the dangerous low-density lipoproteins (LDL) and to some extent account for the health benefits of the Mediterranean diet.

Proteins, which are made up of various combinations of some 22 amino acids, are both animal and vegetable in origin. Most any animal protein provides all the amino acids; it requires a variety of vegetables to do the same. However, a well-balanced meatless diet can do it—as any assiduous vegetarian will attest. Proteins are the tissue-building blocks and a basic dietary component.

Carbohydrates can be both simple (sugars, for instance) and complex (starches as in fruits, vegetables, and grains). Carbohydrates are our energy source. Sugars are considered empty calories, since they provide nothing but energy, have no nutritional value, and, taken in excess (as we now mainly do), contribute to malnutrition by displacing other and better nutrients. They also allow us to store the fat in our diet. Complex carbohydrates, on the other hand, not only require energy consumption to release their energy but contain many other nutrients.

The bottom line: Your daily 2,300-calorie intake should be 25–30 percent fat—mainly unsaturated, 25 percent protein, about 10 percent of it animal in origin—and all the rest of our intake, roughly 50 percent, should be carbohydrates, largely from the complex family. Now, no one should have to sit down, figure out, and total up these components every day. A well-balanced diet based upon the food pyramid (see page 79) will lead you to that goal without any extensive monitoring. We will flesh out these basic recommendations further in a moment.

So, ladies—start your enzymes! Here is your daily bread!

- Remember your basic mix—roughly 50 percent carbohydrates, 25 percent protein, and 25 percent fat—all in the categories that we have covered.

- In the new order of things, dairy products, fats, oils, and sweets are largely relegated to the "treat" level.

- Complex carbohydrates, such as rice, pasta, whole grains, cereals, and so forth, are preferred. Limit refined sugar, syrups, candy, and so on, as much as possible, as well as any other "empty" carbohydrates with no nutritional value. They should go to the "treat" room.

- Fats, although an important dietary component, need to be limited and should contain little cholesterol or other saturated fats. Polyunsaturated and monounsaturated fats are what you are looking for. Olive and canola are the vegetable oils that should be favored for cooking as well as in sauces and dressings. Read labels. You may get some shocks.

•More of your protein should begin to come from vegetables, legumes, and other plant sources.

So, we are looking at a daily ration of:

•three to five portions from vegetables and two to four from fruits

•six to eleven portions from whole grains and cereals, which include breads, rice, pasta, corn, and even potatoes

•two portions of lean animal protein and two from dairy products

Selecting your diet according to these guidelines will provide you with all the essential food elements you need to achieve nutritional balance during your pregnancy and for your lifetime. Moreover, it will provide an adequate **fiber** intake, which we now realize is of great importance in maintaining your general long-term health. Such a diet will also provide most—but not all—of the vitamins and minerals your body requires each day. Unfortunately, studies show that few of us follow anything close to this nutritional pattern. Indeed, the average American diet seems to consist of a soft drink for breakfast, a hamburger with fries and another soft drink for lunch, a TV dinner in the evening—all meals laced and interspersed with coffee. And how many push-ups does a Snickers bar take? This won't do for a healthy body, and especially not for a healthy pregnancy.

Some Other Intake Thoughts

Fluids. We agreed earlier that an adequate intake of fluids is very important at any time, but more so during pregnancy. Fluid needs are increased during pregnancy because of a higher metabolic need as well as an ever-increasing skin surface through which to lose water by evaporation. Restrict coffee because caffeine is a diuretic and thus helps wash water out of your body. Decaf may be better. Fruit juices are fine fluid sources, but watch the calories. Soft drinks, unless sugar-free, also increase caloric intake but are otherwise helpful if they are also caffeine-free. Soft drinks also contain sodium (soda pop—remember?), which may contribute to fluid retention and swelling. Now, take all those things out of soda pop and you are left with colored water! Bottom line: You should drink at least eight glasses of fluids each day—mostly water.

Cow's milk. This liquid is a reasonable source of protein and calcium if it is skimmed totally free of fat and you can digest lactose (milk sugar) without gas or other intestinal problems. (Many people are lactose-intolerant.)

Milk is the "perfect" food only for infants up to two years of age. If you do not drink milk, you must get the proteins, calcium, and fluids from other and safer sources (fat-free yogurt, for instance, which bothers only people with milk protein allergies). Recently the cow's milk that is used in baby formula and that our children keep drinking in subsequent years has also been incriminated as the likely foreign protein trigger for early-onset diabetes! Sounds incredible, but the research work is very believable, even though hotly disputed.

Other Dairy Products. Besides milk, potentially problematic dairy products include butter, eggs, and cheese. Although highly recommended in most pregnancy diets, these substances contain excessive amounts of animal fats and need to be somewhat restricted. Substitute margarine for butter, but only margarine with no cholesterol and less than two grams of saturated fat per tablespoon. Low-fat cottage cheese is acceptable if it also follows the margarine guidelines. Many other low-fat or no-fat cheeses are now in your supermarkets. Egg whites are a perfect source of animal protein. The egg yolk, however, is another matter. It is full of cholesterol and other animal fats. Believe it or not, you can make a marvelous omelet with egg whites, especially if you season it with sage, rosemary or basil, pepper, a little salt, and some creative ingredients like sautéed mushrooms, onions, tomatoes, shrimp, fake crabmeat—and on and on. Or you can use frozen egg substitutes, which are mainly egg whites with some color added. And incidentally, you can now buy fat-free, cholesterol-free cream substitutes that taste really good and can be used with skim milk to make creamy custards, vichyssoise, and many other great unrich but rich-tasting dishes. For example, you can buy fat-free, sugar-free vanilla instant custard, mix it with skim milk with cream substitute in equal parts, and voilà—with some fresh fruit in it you have a great dessert with zip fat, zip cholesterol, and a precious few calories arising only from the skim milk and the fruit. Try it—you'll like it.

This treatment of dairy products seems somewhat harsh and the benefits are more long-term than short-term. There is no reason why you cannot have a breakfast of, say, an egg omelet and buttered toast as an occasional treat.

Salt (sodium). Let's face it: Americans oversalt everything. We generally consume 100 times our actual daily need. Fortunately, our kidneys get rid of excess salt very efficiently under normal circumstances. Salt used to be restricted drastically during pregnancy mainly because it was thought to be a cause of hypertension of pregnancy. While this is no longer considered true, excess salt consumption is a very bad long-term dietary habit. It very likely increases your risk of hypertension in later years, and it certainly increases fluid retention during pregnancy. Most prepared foods are heavily salted, but low-salt alternatives are now everywhere in your supermarket. Read the labels.

Vitamins and minerals. The diet plan outlined here will supply almost all your vitamin and mineral needs without supplementing. However, there are at least three important exceptions.

- •As noted earlier, most women have inadequate **iron** stores when they enter pregnancy and cannot meet the demands of their growing infant. I would advise iron supplementation even before conceiving (see chapter 10). Supplemental iron is a must except for the very, very rare mother with hemachromatosis—an iron storage disorder that she should already know about.

- •**Folic acid** is another substance that most of us have too little of in our diets. In pregnancy it plays an important role in reducing the risk of open neural tube defects such as spina bifida. It is now recommended that folic acid be taken prior to conception, and it is generally included in most vitamin supplements. Folic acid will soon be included in certain foods, such as breads.

- •**Calcium.** We are all deficient in our calcium intake for most of our lives. Cow's milk has long been considered the best source of extra calcium, but for us nonbelievers, there are better ways to get it.

All prenatal vitamin/mineral supplements that I have seen on the market contain these three substances, along with many other additional agents. Each tablet, taken daily, supplies the accepted need for folic acid. Some iron-deficient mothers may need extra iron, as determined by their physician. Some may also need extra calcium, which can easily be supplied by any plain calcium carbonate or calcium citrate tablet.

Not many women (pregnant or not) or men (clearly not pregnant) weigh food, measure portions, establish carbohydrate, fat, and protein percentages, total the daily glasses of fluid swallowed, estimate the number of servings from the basic food groups, banish the salt shaker, throw away egg yolks, or take their prenatal supplement pills each and every day. Nevertheless, and despite all these omissions, we seem to muddle through, and maternal as well as fetal health is steadily improving. If you follow the above guidelines as just *guidelines,* and use common dietary sense, eating a balanced and wide variety of foods, your pregnancy should be nutritionally sound and stable. But take your pills *daily!*

I said earlier that money is not the major source of our widespread malnutrition. And it is not. However, some mothers-to-be have difficulty buying proper food in proper amounts and variety. There are a number of programs that can help them.

- •Federal Supplemental Food Program for Women, Infants, and Children (WIC)

- •Aid to Families with Dependent Children (AFDC)

- •Food stamps

- •Local social service agencies

- •County agents, who can put mothers who need help in touch with any of these sources

No amount of pride should prevent you from receiving this help. We are all here to serve and help one another as best we can.

Sometimes special diets are required for certain obstetrical or metabolic disorders. For instance, a rather bland diet may be necessary to manage severe nausea in the early months, and a diabetic or a mother with Crohn's disease (ulcerative colitis) will certainly need special foods. These and other special dietary problems are best managed by your own obstetrician, perhaps in conjunction with other medical sources and a nutritionist.

Things That Go Bump in the Night

A baby is a living organism from the moment of conception. As we have seen, shortly after a fertilized egg embeds in the womb, it begins to organize into recognizable structures, and once it is an established fetus, movements begin in the form of slight muscular contractions. This occurs sometime in the second month of pregnancy. Such movements soon become more active and more powerful. However, the baby is so small and so well cushioned in your uterus, so completely surrounded by its water bed, that it is usually not until sometime toward the end of the fourth month that movements are first felt. Please make a note of that time, since it may be an important milestone far down the road. There is some variation in this time, and you should not be upset if movements are felt earlier or later. The fetus's movements may be felt only lightly during the whole pregnancy and yet a perfectly normal, angelic child is delivered. Some kick like mules, and you end up with a defensive tackle. Some kick most all of the night, and you end up with an obstetrician in the family. It is clear, then, that some babies are very active and some are not. But the degree of regular movement has only a partial bearing on your baby's actual health.

Sometimes your baby may seem to have stopped moving altogether. The reasons for this loss of awareness of fetal activity are unknown, but in almost all instances, customary movements begin again spontaneously after a while and the pregnancy goes on. You should, however, reassure yourself by going to the doctor's office and having a listen.

At times you may notice a rhythmic tapping inside your abdomen. This sort of movement is caused, we think, by contractions of the fetal diaphragm as it makes slight, preliminary breathing efforts, similar to what happens when we hiccup.

Fetal movements are at first very faint and can best be described as a fluttering or shimmering sensation in the lower abdomen. Many times what are actually fetal movements are thought by the mother to be gas bubbles. After you have once experienced fetal movements, it is easier to recognize them. Usually, then, you are able to feel your baby moving earlier during your second pregnancy than in your first.

Your baby may seem to be everywhere at one time, kicking your ribs and bladder simultaneously. How come? Well, your child is weightless inside you, like an astronaut in space or as you would be in saltwater. A baby can extend all four extremities and its head at the same time—and often does. So it is bump and grind everywhere.

Frequently mothers ask, "Why is it that babies seem to become more active at night?" True, they can pound on your bladder, put a foot into your ribs, hit your mate, and so on, the whole blessed night long. Well, baby does have short, regular sleep and wake periods and thus often appears more active in the evening hours when you are less active. After all, what difference does it make to your precious cargo whether it is night or day? Its home is blacked-out all the time. And so it goes.

Some obstetricians are now asking mothers in certain high-risk pregnancies to monitor their baby's movements during these active periods and to keep records of the activity rate. Under these circumstances, movements should be noted and charted carefully, and any continuing reduction in activity needs to be reported as directed. This information is undoubtedly of real value in assessing fetal well-being in certain high-risk situations. It is true—and we shall explore this later—that there are now many other technical ways to assess fetal well-being, but sometimes these maternal observations still beat them all.

Finally, fetal movements usually diminish shortly after labor begins. After all, it is getting pretty tight inside. If you notice this, do not become alarmed—unless, of course, you are monitoring the activity rate for special reasons, as already noted. Generally, however, a great deal of fetal activity during labor is not a reassuring event, and careful monitoring is important.

Sex

Sex remains the single greatest and most gratifying form of interpersonal communication ever developed. This situation is not likely to change. Pregnancy does nothing to diminish this fact, but it may alter some of the circumstances and some of the ground rules. Here, in a question-and-answer format, are replies to many of your queries about sex during pregnancy.

Is sexual intercourse permitted during pregnancy?
Like breathing and eating, sleeping and awakening, sexual intercourse is not only permissible but desirable during normal pregnancy. The only times it should not be part of your pregnant life are when you don't want to; when certain conditions, which we will go over, make it dangerous; and finally, when it is no longer mutually rewarding. Being philosophical for the moment, I hope your sexual goal has always been to give love to one another rather than just receive it, to respect one another's sexual wishes, and to make love rather than just "doing it." I also hope that you have been able to explore each other's sexual anatomy and, through experimentation and mutual giving, have learned that the more you practice, the better music you make. It is very important during the course of pregnancy, with all its emotional and physical changes, that these sexual aims be continued, further explored, and mutually respected. There are no other terms of endearment here.

How long is sexual intercourse permissible?
Actually, you are asking how long is vaginal penetration permissible. Vaginal penetration is often the culmination of the sexual act and plays a major role in most sexual encounters. Vaginal penetration may occur as long as it is mutually desirable and not painful, and as long as it is not restricted specifically by your physician. Don't call checkmate because of the calendar or clock.

When is intercourse medically not permissible?
Generally, sexual intercourse (vaginal penetration) is restricted when vaginal bleeding is occurring at any stage of pregnancy; when, for whatever reason, there is severe vaginal infection that produces significant pain; when there is a history of incompetent cervical closure (see page 233); when there is a history of premature labor and certain other high-risk situations; when the membranes have ruptured; or when you are in labor. Finally, your doctor may restrict sexual congress for other pertinent reasons that should be made very clear to you.

What may happen to make sex unenjoyable to me?
Physically, you may be subject to local infections in the vagina or to swelling in the vagina and pelvis, particularly late in pregnancy and especially if your baby's head or presenting part is deep in your pelvis. At such times, other forms of mutual gratification can be explored. Emotionally, there are times when fatigue, general discomfort, and other

sensations make sexual activity less than enjoyable. During those times, togetherness, cuddling, and understanding are enough.

After I have a climax, I notice menstrual-type cramping that may last for an hour or so. Why does this happen? Is it dangerous?
When you have an orgasm, your pituitary gland releases a hormone substance that makes your uterus contract. This is almost always the source of your cramping, which is of no danger to you or your pregnancy if none of the abnormalities described earlier exist.

Will such cramps start labor?
Almost never. If they did, a few of us would not be here!

What position is the best for having sexual intercourse while I am pregnant?
Like riding a camel, there is no best position. There are only comfortable and mutually rewarding and satisfying positions. In early pregnancy, there is very little change in your personal sexual habits and positions. As the baby begins to occupy more of your abdomen, you will certainly want to experiment with positions that produce less abdominal pressure. Although such pressure is not necessarily harmful, it is neither rewarding nor pleasant. Other positions to be explored include sitting on top or having him penetrate you from behind. Do what feels comfortable.

Do any special preparations have to be made before having sex during pregnancy?
Sex is usually not prepared for very far in advance, which may be why you have to read this book now. Anyway, spontaneous lovemaking is generally more desirable—but I don't have to tell you that. However, local perineal hygiene with soap and water while showering should be a warm-up event. Local powders, perfumes, and sprays have irritative problems of their own, and douching is not permissible. KY jelly is a safe, water-soluble lubricant, but there are scented lubricants that may be preferred. Sometimes these scented love potions can be irritating to one or both and in a variety of places.

Incidentally, your lover's personal hygiene is very important, since many vaginal infections during pregnancy are transmitted from his fingers, penis, or mouth. Last but not least, in your sexual preparations, take the phone off the hook, lock the door, put the garage door down, sedate the kids, and turn off the TV.

If vaginal penetration is uncomfortable because of pressure or irritation, are there alternatives we may use?
The most common alternatives are oral and anal intercourse or mutual masturbation. Again, if oral-genital relationships are desirable, personal hygiene is of vast importance.

Insofar as anal intercourse is concerned, if vaginal penetration is uncomfortable at this stage, it is more than likely that anal penetration will be even more so. Also, anal penetration followed by vaginal penetration is out during pregnancy, as the risk of subsequent vaginal infection is too great. Late in pregnancy, mutual masturbation may be the only alternative. One more thing: blowing into the vagina, a not uncommon sexual practice, is far too dangerous at this time.

I have a constant discharge from my breasts during pregnancy, which you have called colostrum, and this increases during sexual activity when my husband fondles and suckles my breasts. Is this harmful?
No, but the secretions may be bitter, and he may wish to change this form of breast stimulation. He cannot hurt your nipples unless he bites them or has an oral infection. Incidentally, it is important to keep your nipples soft, supple, and everted if you plan to nurse your baby. Sexual stimulation will help this process, and at other times you will want to massage and oil your nipples, gently tugging them outwards as you do.

Will sex make the water break?
In a normal pregnancy, no. When the cervix begins to open prematurely, however, in the condition called cervical incompetence (see page 233), sexual activity may rupture the membranes. You and your physician will be aware of this condition, and vaginal penetration will be off limits.

Will my climax change during pregnancy?
Your sexual drive is highly involved in your emotional life and subject to vast changes under the psychological stress as well as hormonal changes of pregnancy.
Therefore, you may have a deeper or more recurrent climax, a less sustained climax, or even none at all. If serious orgasmic failure occurs during pregnancy and continues afterward for any sustained time, it is important to seek counseling. This situation is almost always reversible.

Will his desires change?
They may. He, too, may have some emotional remodeling related to the pregnancy, which may be both good and bad. For instance, he may wish to overprotect you; he may fear the pregnancy; he may not want the changes that the baby produces in your body and in your daily and sexual lifestyle. There may be a thousand other subconscious factors that interfere with his normal sexual drive. He needs to talk with you about them—if, indeed, he realizes them.

If he and I develop a significant sexual problem during pregnancy or afterward, how can we best cope with this problem?
A serious sexual problem is not likely to arise if you have communicated freely as a couple in the past and have had no hangups or other communication problems during the pregnancy. However, should a sexual problem of significant magnitude occur while you are pregnant, there are resources available to help you cope. First, of course, discuss the difficulty with your partner. Should this avenue fail or not be open to you, you should next talk with your obstetrician. Only a few doctors are trained to manage these problems themselves, and usually, in a busy practice, they also do not have the time to explore them with you in sufficient depth. However, if yours is a patient-oriented doctor trained in sexual counseling (and they are on the increase), you may be able to get sufficient help without going any further. Otherwise, you should ask your doctor to refer you to a good counselor. There are many good sex therapists and clinical psychologists available.

Showing

Somewhere between the third and fifth months, your waistline, which may have already eased just a bit, will begin to expand noticeably, and the flatland below it will be replaced with a perceptible and visible bulge.

This anatomical phenomenon is known as showing. For numerous reasons, it occurs at different times in different women. The abdomen of a mother who has previously borne children stretches more readily, so that she is more likely to show early in her pregnancy. Also, basic anatomy makes a difference. For instance, women with long, deep abdomens may hardly show at all during pregnancy. The size of the uterus is another controlling factor. This, in turn, depends on the baby's weight, the number of babies present, and the amount of surrounding amniotic fluid.

All these factors plus a few others contribute to determining when you lose the battle of the bulge. And whenever this might be, it has no bearing on whether your pregnancy is normal, massive, misdated, or multiple. All it determines is when you have to get out of slacks and into sacks!

A Simple Matter of Elimination

Constipation
We spend the early years of our children's lives training them to hold on to things until we can get them on the potty. They spend the rest of their

years trying to get on the potty when it is convenient rather than when the urge comes. The result of this constant colonic conflict is constipation and the sale of millions of dollars' worth of laxatives, enemas, and hemorrhoid preparations.

Constipation, a prevalent problem in our society, is even more common during pregnancy. Functional changes in the intestines as well as pressure on the lower bowel and rectum invite constipation, and even worse, the tendency toward constipation combined with rectal pressure predisposes you to the formation of hemorrhoids, which lead to rectal burning, itching, pain, and bleeding. Clearly, constipation should be avoided by:

- establishing a regular morning or evening bathroom ritual

- immediate responding (when humanly possible) to the desire to have a bowel movement

- eating fruits, raw or cooked, that have a laxative effect

- eating roughage and high-fiber foods such as leafy vegetables and prepared cereals, particularly bran and other high-fiber cereals and foods

- drinking plenty of fluids

- engaging in meaningful, regular exercise

Having regular, soft bowel movements helps greatly in the prevention of hemorrhoids. It is important to avoid straining after the initial bowel evacuation, even if you feel there is more material to be passed. This feeling of fullness may well be due to engorgement of the rectal veins, and straining only engorges them further, bringing them to the outside and producing clinical hemorrhoids. The treatment of hemorrhoids, when they do occur, should be individualized, and you should call your doctor for proper care.

You may sometimes have to resort to laxatives during pregnancy. There are several categories of laxatives—some safe, some not so safe.

- The most common and safest laxative to start with is the **bulking agents** that are capable of softening the stool mass. They sometimes cause abdominal bloating and gas but are usually the gentlest, least irritating of all agents. Examples are bran, methyl cellulose, and psyllium derivatives.

- **Stimulant laxatives**, which consist of aloes, cascara, and, until recently, phenolphthalein, work directly on the colon and, when used frequently or for a long time, can permanently damage that part of the intestines.

- **Saline laxatives** such as milk of magnesia and magnesium citrate induce water secretion into the bowel and thus soften the stool. They should never be used chronically.

- Finally, **emollients,** which include dioctyl sodium sulfosuccinate and mineral oil, allow water within the bowel to enter the stool mass. These laxatives are usually quite safe.

- Prepackaged **enemas** and **suppositories** of saline-type laxatives can be used occasionally and are safer than some of the other laxatives.

Your physician should be made aware of a significant constipation problem. He or she will surely offer help in selecting which program or laxative is proper for you and will follow your progress with you.

Incidentally, the iron in your prenatal vitamin/mineral supplement may produce a black bowel movement that is constipating. You may have to get your iron some other way. Ask your doctor. More rarely, iron will give you diarrhea and, again, will have to be taken in another form.

Habits

Good habits are proper eating and sleeping, regular exercise, scrupulous personal hygiene, responsible living, speaking the truth, driving properly, and so on. Bad habits are what we are saddled with, sometimes constitute our way of life, and often lead us on an addictive hunt for what we do not really want. We are all creatures of habit, and generally your habits—both good and bad—will have been well formed by the time you conceive. Most bad habits affect pregnancy, although a few do not.

Among our worst bad habits—and those that seriously compromise pregnancy and our children—are substance abuses. Despite the vast outpouring of warning information in every conceivable media source, 6 percent of pregnant mothers continue to use illicit drugs, 20 percent continue to drink alcohol, and another 20 percent smoke tobacco! These incredible, but reliable, figures are fearsome—not only because of their impact on pregnancy and the suffering babes but because of what they tell us about ourselves and where we are headed. In the past, our ignorance about the destructive impact of these habits could account for their continuance among pregnant mothers, but knowing what we all now know, it is hard to reconcile these figures with motherhood at any level.

Tobacco

Although tobacco use is steadily declining, the largest decline is among older citizens. Among women of childbearing age, there are 3,000 new smokers each day. Here are most of the known effects of the drugs in tobacco upon pregnancy, childbirth, and the newborn:

• Newborn birth weight is low. The more cigarettes the mother smokes, the smaller the infant and the greater the risk for prematurity.

• The risk of preterm labor is increased.

• Abnormal bleeding late in pregnancy is more common among women who smoke. This bleeding is generally related to placental separation or its abnormal and dangerous location.

• The infant is born nicotine-addicted and suffers withdrawal after birth. Later on the child is slow to develop, has a lower IQ score, and may suffer from reading disorders as well as conduct disorders.

• Exposed to passive smoke after birth, the child will have respiratory infections, bronchitis, ear problems, and asthma at a significantly increased rate. The risk of sudden infant death syndrome (SIDS) is also greater.

• Of course, the smoking mother is at increased risk for chronic obstructive lung disorders, cardiovascular disease and stroke, peptic ulcer disease, cancer of the lungs, bladder, cervix, and breast, and a greatly foreshortened, restricted life.

• Mothers exposed to passive smoking are equally at risk for fetal damage and, as the airline attendants recently demonstrated in court, are at great risk from tobacco's 1,000 diverse and poisonous chemicals.

Unfortunately, some heavily nicotine-addicted mothers need more than this sad but certain litany as they struggle with their immense problem. What options are available for those seeking help with nicotine addiction?

• The Fagerstrom Test for Nicotine Dependence is a six-question test designed to measure the degree of addiction and thus distinguish between those smokers who can attempt personal and private cessation and those requiring intervention help. The test was first published in 1991 in the *British Journal of Addiction* but has been widely published and made available in this country.

• Group or private therapy is readily available for those who are more highly addicted.

• A recent study indicates that nicotine skin patches may be safe to use sparingly during pregnancy. No adverse fetal effects were observed, but the study is preliminary and will need more confirmation. Nicotine from the patches does, of course, enter the bloodstream. That's how they work. The blood levels were, however, lower than those produced by smoking.

•Passive smoking in a pregnant mother's household should be eliminated. If those you live with cannot or will not quit, they must smoke elsewhere. We have read about or seen the damage of passive smoke, but remember that passive smoke may also prompt an ex-smoker to restart. Passive smoking is thankfully disappearing from public places. Pregnant women exposed to smoking in their workplace can have it stopped by appealing to the local Occupational Safety and Health Administration (OSHA) office.

If you are having difficulty with this problem, here are two more suggestions.

•Have an ultrasound done early in your pregnancy and watch your little one moving about within you. Besides yourself, you are damaging this struggling innocent babe.

•Ask your doctor to draw a carbon monoxide blood level from you. Compare it to what it should be. (It should be zip.)

A sad reminder to end this addictive trail: only one-third of pregnant women who smoke will stop during pregnancy, and of those who do stop, 70 percent restart during the following year.

In case you were wondering, I have been, for 25 years, an arrested nicotine addict.

Alcohol

Although less addictive than tobacco, alcohol nevertheless is a major social and health problem that affects almost every household somewhat. Its effect upon pregnancy can be disastrous.

Here are some points for you concerning alcohol and pregnancy.

•Ethanol (the active agent in liquor) freely crosses the placenta and enters your baby's circulation.

•The fetal danger is greatest in the first trimester, but brain damage continues and increases throughout pregnancy.

•Fetal alcohol syndrome (FAS) has three major components— growth retardation, facial abnormalities, and central nervous system dysfunctions.

• Obstetrical problems include early spontaneous abortion and intrauterine fetal death.

• Paternal alcohol intake has a lesser but nevertheless real chance of inducing FAS by damage that sperm sustain from alcohol.

• FAS babies face alcohol withdrawal symptoms at birth that can be life-threatening.

A chronic alcoholic presents a disastrous picture during pregnancy. According to a recent study, she has a 45–50 percent chance of producing a severely malformed infant. Because of this risk of congenital malformation and all the other associated dangers, a chronic alcoholic should avoid pregnancy; if it takes place, therapeutic abortion should be seriously considered. In many practicing obstetricians' opinion, this sad disease is in fact a good, sufficient, and compelling reason for an abortion.

Although a glass of wine with dinner after the third month will probably have no harmful fetal or obstetrical effect, the arguments against alcohol during pregnancy are so compelling that no physician (and that includes this writer) is prepared to condone any alcohol ingestion whatsoever for the total duration. By the way, that admonition includes some alcohol-based cough syrups and tonics—read all labels!

In case you were wondering, I have wine with my two main meals each and every day.

Marijuana

There has been no significant research on the effects of tetrahydrocannabinol (marijuana's active ingredient) on pregnancy or the fetus. The reason seems obvious—pregnant users don't wish to make their habit known to researchers. Thus, not much is known about its pregnancy-damaging potential.

Cocaine

With the advent of "crack," an inexpensive, easily obtained, and stable derivative of cocaine, widespread use followed. There are at least 10 million occasional and 5 million habitual users. In women, users are concentrated in the reproductive age group. Significantly more research is available involving cocaine users because they are more readily identifiable in clinic settings. Disregarding the massive, often fatal maternal risks from cocaine, its harmful pregnancy effects are multiple.

- •Spontaneous abortion and fetal death in utero are common.

- •Premature rupture of the membranes, premature labor, intrauterine growth retardation, premature placental separation are all frequent consequences.

- •The teratogenic effects of cocaine are unknown, but microcephaly (small head), limb reduction, and genito-urinary deformities are all regular possibilities.

Heroin

For a number of reasons, heroin use is on the rise. The obstetrical and fetal risks of heroin mirror those of cocaine, plus one even more deadly for the fetus. Newborn infants of heroin-addicted mothers risk severe narcotic withdrawal and even death if it goes undiagnosed. Moreover, methadone, which is used to manage heroin addicts attempting withdrawal, can itself produce withdrawal crises in the newborn.

"Ice" and LSD

Research on the use of amphetamines (ice) and LSD, while relatively common, is limited. Generally ice mimics cocaine in its pregnancy and fetal effects. Even less is known about LSD—which was once thought to inflict chromosomal damage, a problem that can no longer be attributed to it.

Our lack of firm documentation of the risks these agents impose does not mean that they are safe or acceptable during pregnancy or at any time. It simply represents the gaps in our knowledge about them.

The point of this section on drug abuse is not to moralize but to advise—mainly on what these agents do to an uninvolved but soon-to-be-involved infant. The rest is up to you. Your habits are your own business—but so is birthing a healthy infant.

Caffeine: A Bit Player

We get caffeine from coffee, tea, cocoa, and cola drinks, and thus we all get a lot of caffeine daily, one way or another. Numerous studies have been undertaken to rule out caffeine as a harmful drug in pregnancy. In spite of all this work, there is still no absolutely clear answer. It has been implicated as a cause of spontaneous abortion and intrauterine growth retardation, but the final proof is not there. All we know is that very heavy consumption does indeed lead to IUGR. Those who have studied the drug most thoroughly say that up to 300 milligrams (three good and full coffee cups) daily appears to be a safe load.

Long Time No Z's

Sleep is a natural physiological function. Yet for whatever reason, one-third of all adults have sleep problems and physicians write about 55,000 prescriptions for sleeping pills *each and every day*—or night. Insomnia, a major disorder of our civilization, is being studied more deeply all the time. Sleep labs are popping up all over the country, and treatment clinics are available in most large cities, which is where most insomnia is found.

Whatever your sleeping habits have been, pregnancy has a major impact on them, an impact that begins almost as soon as the pregnancy does. Thus, in the days shortly following conception, it becomes evident that the mother-to-be is very sleepy most of the time. This drowsy state, mentioned before as an early symptom of pregnancy, will disappear as the middle months come along. Until it does, give in to it and sleep. Insomnia is thus rarely a complication of early pregnancy.

Later pregnancy is a different matter. Many things will try to rob you of sleep in the months ahead, such as:

- increased body metabolism producing increased body heat awareness

- increased pressure from within your abdomen, both above and below

- frequent need to empty your bladder

- general discomfort and inability to find and stay in a comfortable sleeping position

- regurgitation of stomach contents with the resultant heartburn

- unpleasant dreams

- a noisy bed partner

This is a disturbing and formidable list, but you may not have to cope with all of these problems. Nevertheless, sleep is a very precious commodity as term approaches and is beset, as you can see, by a number of blockades. Here are some helpful hints:

- Use your bed only to sleep—or for lovemaking. Don't read, rest, or watch TV in bed. If you have a medical problem requiring rest (such as hypertension), use a sofa or couch in another room and avoid your bed if possible. Also, you could try some of your old lovemaking spots instead of the bed. Remember?

- If you take a nap, be sure to do so early in the day.

•Eliminate background noise as much as possible or mask such noises with wash-out or white sound. Tapes of such sounds (rain, seashore, and so on) are available everywhere. Sometimes a room fan provides the desired soothing effect.

•Avoid caffeine substances after 4:00 P.M., and cut down on all fluids before bedtime.

•If you have heartburn and you regurgitate, don't eat before bedtime, keep recommended antacids at hand, and try sleeping semi-propped up. Cracked ice is a safe but temporary cure for heartburn. Unfortunately, it melts and eventually has to go somewhere, and your bladder sooner or later advises you of where that place is.

•A waterbed, foam rubber, or air mattress may provide you with more comfort.

•Focus on a boring task, such as counting sheep—or better still, on planning a happy future event.

•Have a very close friend give you a gentle massage. And get him an anti-snoring nasal strip!

Sedatives and sleeping pills are not recommended during pregnancy.

To Sleep—Perchance to Dream

Dreaming, which occurs during light sleep periods, is often greatly enhanced during pregnancy, which features more light sleep. Unpleasant dreams, unfortunately, are also more common. Such dreams often center on bad pregnancy outcomes. It may reassure you to know that these dreams, unfortunate and frightening as they may be, bear no relationship to the health or outcome of your pregnancy. There is no effective way to abolish these dreams. Sharing them with someone right away will ease their impact, and they will be gone after delivery—when you'll be dreaming instead about an uninterrupted good night's sleep!

More Pregnant Pauses

•Consider this dietary advice, which was given to pregnant women about a hundred years ago.
  Eat only *twice* daily . . . excessive indulgence in food has hurried more people to the grave than war, famine, pestilence, and alcohol

combined . . . its ravages are ceaseless; from year to year it pursues its work of destruction without pause for interruption. . . . It wastes not only cities and provinces but rioting throughout the whole broad world, it spreads disease and death amongst all classes, ages, sexes, and conditions—maidens and matrons—infants and children—the feeble and robust—all are swept indiscriminately into the grave by this fell destroyer. (Wilhelmine D. Schott, *Health Hints to Women* [New York: Charles P. Somerby, 1883], p. 87)

• An improper diet is actually more dangerous to your baby than moderate smoking and drinking! But all of them are harmful.

• Since about 11,000 babies are born each day in the United States, it follows that at least that many, and certainly more, pregnancies occur each day—or night. Then, if the nausea of early pregnancy exists in about half of these conceptions and lasts for about three months, you can see that there must be some 5 million sufferers out there at any one time! Not too comforting a thought, although misery loves company.

• Between 1991 and 1995 (the latest year for collected statistics), the rate of high alcohol consumption among pregnant women *quadrupled!* This figure is based on a study of some 33,000 women between the ages of 18 and 44 conducted by the Centers for Disease Control (CDC).

• The popular press has falsely reported that the nausea and vomiting of early pregnancy is a protective mechanism. It supposedly keeps women from eating certain pungent and bitter vegetables that could be harmful to their pregnancy. These foods included broccoli, brussels sprouts, spinach, peppers, cabbage, cauliflower, garlic, and potatoes. That report belongs where two-week-old vegetable leftovers belong—in the garbage or the compost.

Diary

My Third Month

Problems_____

Medications_____

_____

_____

Travel_____

_____

_____

Diet Problems_____

_____

_____

Baby moved? When?_____

_____

What's going on in the world?_____

_____

_____

_____

What's going on in my life?_____

_____

_____

_____

My thoughts and feelings_____

_____

_____

_____

Doctor's appointment_____

_____

_____

Questions to ask_____

_____

_____

_____

_____

_____

_____

_____

_____

_____

_____

_____

_____

_____

_____

_____

_____

_____

_____

_____

_____

_____

_____

_____

_____

_____

_____

_____

_____

Four

My Fourth Lunar Month

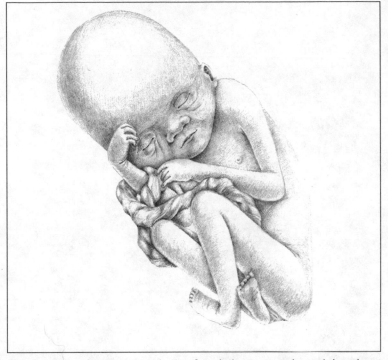

The fetus inside you, now in its fourth lunar month, weighs about three ounces (85 grams) and is some six and one half inches (16 centimeters) in length. It is moving actively and you should know it. Although completely formed, your baby-in-the-making can still be damaged by a large number of unusual substances and activities, most all of which will be covered as we move along.

On ultrasound, it is now becoming difficult to visualize the whole fetus in one frame. As growth continues, it becomes necessary to take multiple pictures to visualize all we need to see. Thus, at full term, as many as 15 frames may be required. This ultrasound captures as much of a normal 16-week fetus as possible.

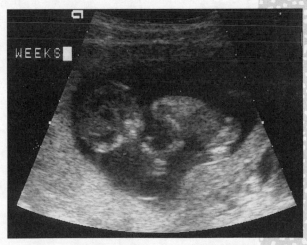

The fourth lunar month is a rather quiet time in your pregnancy—rather like the eye of a hurricane! After all, your energy is returning, food looks great again, your passenger is not taking up enough room to really matter, and you can still get into your jeans—a little snug, maybe, but they zip. You are moving on, however, and when you finally do leave the serene eye of this pregnant hurricane, you are going to be swept on rather quickly—fortunately, to somewhere you want to go, and hopefully without too much turbulence!

This relatively peaceful spell will give us time to talk about some disorders that can complicate pregnancy. Although a significant number of these disorders are not very pleasant and may never involve you, we need to deal with them just in case. You may wonder, after reading about some of them, how any child could reach this earth safely, undamaged, in good health, and perfectly formed. But nature, with its marvelous ability to overprotect, scan, and adapt, guards your baby much better than you could ever imagine. Even so, nature does not always do what we consider is best or what pleases us.

Vaginal Secretions

Vaginal secretions are normally somewhat acidic and are made up of:

- mucous secreted by the cervix

- a clear liquid transudate that regularly flows across the vaginal lining

- superficial skin cells that exfoliate (break away) by the billions from the constantly growing vaginal epithelium (skin)

- bacteria (*Lactobacillus*) that normally colonize the vagina and are necessary for vaginal hygiene and health

- lactic acid (normal vaginal epithelium cells are rich in glycogen [sugar], which bacteria breaks down into lactic acid, thus adding the characteristic odor to vaginal secretions)

Normal, healthy vaginal secretions are increased during pregnancy because of the intense local congestion. Thus, a heavier discharge is not unusual, but its characteristics should be unchanged. Should the secretions become irritating, offensive, painful, or bloody, consult your doctor. Remember, douching must be avoided.

Minor Vaginal Infections

There are three relatively minor vaginal infections to contend with during pregnancy: yeast, trichomonas, and the possibly more problematic bacterial vaginosis (BV).

Yeast

This is the most common vaginal infection of all, and one of the most irritating. Generally there is redness and swelling at the vaginal entrance along with a thick white discharge. If, for some important reason, you need an antibiotic while you are pregnant, you become much more susceptible to a vaginal yeast infection and probably should be prepared for it. Suppositories and creams, now available over-the-counter, are quite effective but cannot prevent a recurrence. Yeast infections can be, and often are, sexually transmitted from your partner's penis, hands, or mouth. However, it is not necessarily a sexually transmitted disease (STD) because the yeast organisms are everywhere—even on your own body—although you are usually resistant to them. To protect yourself from reinfection from any source, put paper around all visited toilet seats; take showers, not tub baths; wear a panty liner; and avoid sex until all symptoms subside. If they recur after sex, you've found your culprit.

Trichomonas

This mild, usually sexually transmitted vaginal infection is caused by a single-cell organism that dwells in and around the vagina and the male prostate gland. When the vagina is involved, there is usually a thin, yellow discharge of unpleasant odor, and there is also usually a good deal of itching and irritation both inside and out. Although in most cases the infection responds readily to a chemical agent called metronidazole, physicians have resisted its use in pregnancy since it is an oral preparation. As time goes on, however, more studies reveal that the drug is apparently safe even in pregnancy, and so it may be possible to use it to treat this infection at any time. You and your physician would have to discuss that option. Certain vaginal suppositories can be helpful. The same preventive hygiene used to avoid yeast infections should be followed. A trichomonas infection has no known effect on pregnancy. Apparently its most serious side effect is on interpersonal relationships: Who brought it home?

Bacterial Vaginosis (BV)

This is a relatively new term coined for a relatively old bacterial STD of the vagina. Previous names included hemophilus vaginitis and Gardnerella vaginitis. The infection is bacterial and accompanied by a moderate watery discharge with a fishy odor. It has been difficult to diagnose accurately in the past, but more sensitive tests now make the diagnosis much easier. Like trichomonas, this infection usually responds to metronidazole. Recent evidence indicates that BV needs to be treated even during pregnancy. It is becoming more and more certain that BV contributes significantly to premature labor. Thus, it is important to screen for it during pregnancy and to treat it. Metronidazole, as noted earlier, apparently poses no danger to the fetus.

This recently discovered connection between BV and risk of premature labor should probably move BV into the major infection camp, but we will leave it here for the moment. No matter where it sits, it needs to be treated.

Major Vaginal Infections

Some serious vaginal infections may complicate pregnancy. Such infections are considered serious because they can damage a fetus as well as its host. Almost all of them are sexually transmitted diseases (STDs). Some are bacterial and some are viral.

Chlamydia

A bacterial infection, this particular sexually transmitted disease has for an initial symptom only a mildly irritating, usually yellowish discharge. Often the discharge goes unnoticed and, in the nonpregnant state, can silently move up from the vagina and produce tubal closure, pelvic inflammatory disease, and thus sterility, along with many other pelvic problems. Chlamydia is also implicated in premature rupture of the membranes and premature labor. Two-thirds of the babies born to infected mothers contract the infection during vaginal delivery and are at risk for severe eye, throat, and lung disease—even sudden infant death syndrome (SIDS) later on. The present chlamydia epidemic is said to involve up to 40 percent of women of childbearing age, with 4 million new cases each year!

Fortunately, tests are now available for chlamydia, making the diagnosis easier and more certain. Appropriate antibiotics can safely be given during pregnancy.

Gonorrhea

Once a popular pelvic passenger, this bacteria-caused STD is losing ground to the newer infections. Yes, it is still spreading (particularly newer, more resistant mutant forms), but it is not spreading as fast as the newer STDs. The discharge from gonorrhea is usually heavy, yellow, and irritating. It can be cultured easily and treated with appropriate antibiotics—to which, as mentioned, it becomes more resistant all the time. The antibiotics can and must be used during pregnancy. Infants delivered vaginally in the presence of gonorrhea risk permanent blindness if not treated at once. Most states have laws mandating that all newborns' eyes receive treatment drops in the event that the mother has undetected gonorrhea.

Mycoplasmosis

This is a less common STD that is virtually symptom-free. It is usually discovered in an infertility workup by blood testing, since it is virtually impossible to culture in most clinical settings. Besides infertility, its main effect on pregnancy is its involvement in repeated miscarriages—which is why infertility specialists usually discover it. It is treated with specific antibiotics, and the results may be followed by regular blood testing.

Beta Hemolytic Streptococcus (GBS)

GBS is a common disease-causing bacteria found in many other parts of the body as well as the vagina. Whether it is sexually transmitted or not is still uncertain, but it most likely is not. Beta strep can be found in up to 40 percent of all vaginal cultures, and it poses no threat whatsoever— except in pregnancy. It is implicated as but one more cause of premature rupture of the membranes. Further, pregnant women can transmit the infection to their unborn fetus or, at birth, to their newborn. This may create no problem, but sometimes the infant can become severely ill. Moreover, GBS can be transmitted to the newborn for some time after birth.

GBS is usually symptom-free, and therefore it is important to test for it. Tests in early pregnancy are usually not useful because the major trouble takes place at the end of pregnancy. Generally it is tested for early in the month preceding delivery, and, if present, appropriate antibiotics are given. Women at risk for GBS should have antibiotics during labor unless recent cultures have been negative. Those at risk include women who are experiencing:

- preterm labor (before 37 weeks)

- premature rupture of the membranes before 37 weeks

•premature rupture of the membranes lasting longer than 18 hours before labor or delivery

•fever during labor

Syphilis

In centuries gone by, syphilis played the role now captured by AIDS. It destroyed king and peasant alike, produced millions of deformed, destroyed infants, and undoubtedly altered the course of history. Columbus brought it from the western hemisphere to the eastern. That doubtful favor was repaid when AIDS was recently given to us by Africa. The advent of penicillin arrested the ravages of syphilis, although it still marches on and is developing an immunity to penicillin and all the newer antibiotics. Syphilis is not strictly a vaginal infection, but it usually starts there in women with a shallow ulcer, painful if on the outside at the entrance, painless, often unnoticed, further inside.

Not too long ago, universal law demanded that a blood test for syphilis be performed on all newborns, all pregnant women, all people entering a hospital (as a patient) for any reason, all people wanting a marriage license, all people entering the armed services, all medical students, all hospital employees, and so forth. Consent was neither required nor sought. You will undoubtedly have a test for syphilis when you have your routine prenatal blood work done. How the world has changed! Imagine trying to do that type of testing for AIDS!

History aside, syphilis is indeed making a great comeback—mainly in large metropolitan areas, but it is moving outward as well. Again, in women, the disease usually starts with a vaginal ulcer (but the original ulcer may also be oral or rectal) that heals very slowly. The ulcers are much larger than those of herpes, and develop a built-up or raised edge. They may not be detected if they start deep in the vagina except that they may produce a heavy yellow discharge from secondary infection. Syphilis soon spreads throughout the entire body; it has disastrous effects on a fetus. We are beginning to see these poor syphilis-infected infants again. Antibiotics are still the treatment of choice for the infected mother but are useless for the damaged baby.

Human Papilloma Virus (HPV)

Here is an STD that is probably even more prevalent than chlamydia. It is a virus that takes up residence in the female vagina and cervix, and on the male penis. It can produce warts called condyloma around and in the vagina and rectum as well as on male genital and rectal areas. In the absence of these warts, HPV has no visible lesions and produces no symptoms. HPV lesions that enter the cervix are the source, sooner or later, of almost all cervical cancer. We are thus seeing a major epidemic of cervical precancer and cancer in the childbearing age group. There are well over 60 identified forms of HPV, but two or three of them are more virulent than all the others and are the source of most serious problems. We now have the ability to determine in the office the particular HPV type with which we are dealing.

The condyloma—or warts—are treated during pregnancy with a variety of chemicals, and in severe, widespread cases by laser surgery. Newborn infants can pick up the virus while being delivered and may, during their first five years of life, develop papillomas on their vocal cords that can be very dangerous to them. Condylomas often grow rapidly during pregnancy and become difficult to treat. Although the virus can become dormant for long intervals, there is no known way, at present, to rid our bodies of it. We can only manage its consequences.

Because of the great risk posed by HPV for cancer of the cervix, it is important that you have regular Pap smears, pregnant or not. There is no other way to screen for precancerous lesions of the cervix, and the Pap smear, with appropriate follow-up and care, represents one of the greatest public health tools ever provided for us. Abnormal precancerous lesions found on the cervix during pregnancy are treated locally in a variety of ways—up to and including coring out (conization) part of the cervix. Cancer of the cervix found at this time must be dealt with on a very individual basis after adequate consultation with a gynecological oncologist.

We have now reviewed the majority of the vaginal infections that may complicate pregnancy. It is easy to see why preventive care is so important. Most of the time any vaginal infection that plagues you will simply be yeast. Nonetheless, do not let it slide.

The TORCH Syndrome

The TORCH syndrome is an acronym for a group of infectious processes all known—or highly suspected—to bring damage to babies in the uterus, at birth, or during their early life. Let's look at the elements of the word.

T—toxoplasmosis

O—others: hepatitis B; B streptococcus; influenza, mumps, and chicken pox (varicella); others as yet unknown

R—rubella (German measles)

C—cytomegalovirus

H—herpes virus II

Many of these infectious processes are mentioned elsewhere in this book. Why, then, are they grouped together here?

- •Infections in newborns associated with these agents are generally indistinguishable except by very special tests.

- •Infection in newborns is often inapparent and late to appear, but it can cause long-term serious damage.

- •Most important, infection in the mother is often clinically not apparent or simply passed off as the flu or mono or "some virus."

- •Treatment is difficult for most of these infections, but prevention and treatment are improving.

- •Grouped together, they represent a significant problem that needs medical and social attention.

- •While it has been estimated that these infections involve as many as 5 to 15 percent of all pregnancies, at most only 1 to 2 percent of the affected fetuses are structurally damaged as a result.

Infants who are afflicted by any one of the TORCH infections may have a variety of abnormalities, depending on when the infection strikes. If it occurs in early pregnancy (the first trimester), the damage generally involves the heart, eyes, neurological system, or blood-forming system. Infections sustained later in the pregnancy generally produce more subtle problems, such as failure to thrive, low birth weight, perceptual handicaps, mental retardation, and certain other more rare conditions.

As noted, taken alone, these infections don't represent a big problem, but grouped together, they are considerably more compelling. Each will be briefly covered here.

Toxoplasmosis

This organism is present in the droppings of cats, which probably originally became diseased by eating infected rodents. Toxoplasmosis is also present in uncooked meat, particularly pork, although this is rare in the United States. And finally, of course, it is in human blood—the blood of those infected by cats or by food.

It is transmitted from these sources by a variety of mechanisms. Symptoms are just like those of the flu or mononucleosis, but toxoplasmosis can cause miscarriages, stillbirths, prematurity, low birth weight for pregnancy duration, and infectious and developmental problems in later life. There are two tests now available for this disease. The first test determines whether you were ever exposed to it by measuring appropriate antibody levels in your blood. The second test determines whether you have had a recent infection that did not alert you with significant symptoms. Apparently, if there is any possibility of exposure, both tests should be given. The FDA has recently cautioned us not to rely on a single test in determining the potential for the presence of toxoplasmosis. The treatment for active infection involves appropriate antibiotics. Preventive care is as follows:

- •Avoid cats. If you own one, do not handle its litter box, whether it is an indoor or an outdoor cat. Don't even let the cat lick your face. Unless you love the cat more than your expected child, lend it to a friend.

- •Cook meat thoroughly.

- •This is probably unnecessary and ridiculous to suggest, but avoid any suggestion of a blood transfusion or blood products unless, of course, it is a life-saving measure.

Your obstetrician probably will test you for toxoplasmosis activity with the appropriate measures when you first see him or her, and with the second test if you should develop a suspicious viral-like infection. Should your baby somehow have a toxoplasmosis problem at or after birth, appropriate treatment is at hand. Remember, in order to infect a baby, all these TORCH infections must cross the placenta. They don't often make it across, so the baby is generally protected. TORCH infections *must be* watched for, though.

Hepatitis B

Approximately 22,000 infants are born annually in our country to mothers who are chronically infected with the hepatitis B virus (HBV). This virus can be transmitted in many ways—for example, by blood transfusion, needle puncture, tattooing, ear piercing, contamination in a hospital, contamination by human feces or blood, and even by sexual intercourse (through contact with contaminated saliva, semen, or feces). The later in pregnancy hepatitis is acquired, the more likely the child is to acquire it and thus possibly become a carrier.

Symptoms may be specific or they may be like any of the others in the TORCH family. Passive immunization can be given, and fortunately a vaccine is available now to protect susceptible and exposed individuals.

Newborn infants of infected mothers must receive immune globulin within 12 hours after birth and be started on a series of vaccinations in the first 24 hours after birth.

Here is a list of potential candidates for acquiring HBV:

•women with hepatitis signs or symptoms

•intravenous drug abusers

•women who have had body piercing or tattoos

•women who are sexually active with a number of partners

•immigrants from Third World countries

•hemodialysis patients or workers

•health care workers exposed to blood or blood products

•women with liver enzyme abnormalities

•women with needle-stick injuries

•women who have had sexual contact with known carriers

•women who work in custodial institutions

The good news—if there is any—is that:

•Adequate testing is available.

•Prenatal testing is almost always done in the United States and is now mandatory in some states.

•A preventive vaccine is widely available and very safe.

Hepatitis C, another liver-infecting virus, has only recently been identified. It is transmitted just as HBV is. Little is known about its pregnancy effects as yet, and there is no vaccine.

Influenza and Mumps

The evidence is uncertain, but growing, that there is a relationship between some influenza and mumps infections and later severe blood disorders in a child exposed within the uterus. Vaccines for both influenza and mumps are available, but only influenza vaccine may be given while pregnancy exists. During pregnancy it is wise to avoid public exposure in epidemic areas. However, if you are teaching school or working in a hospital, what can you do? It is easy to say, "Stay home"—but not always easy to do.

Varicella (Chicken Pox)

This is perhaps the most infectious of all common viral diseases, with a contagion rate of more than 90 percent among all who are exposed. Interestingly, this member of the herpes virus family is in the same large group as herpes virus II, which has been a front-page, somewhat distorted attention-getter in recent times. Chicken pox occurs in only 1 of 7,500 pregnancies, and the diagnosis is usually made by clinical signs on the skin. Although there is some very slight risk of the mother ending up with deadly varicella pneumonia, this catastrophe is fortunately exceedingly rare. The fetal damage if mother does get chicken pox includes skin scarring, small lesions on the extremities, and greatly increased susceptibility to many future infections. No treatment exists for this viral infection. If you have a child or are around kids who have recently been vaccinated, you stand a slight chance of catching the virus (1 in 10,000). This could be a dangerous fetal situation if you happen to be pregnant. However, interestingly, it is less likely to happen than would be the case if the child had developed chicken pox by contagion.

Rubella (German Measles)

This disease could be wiped from the face of the earth, just as smallpox has been and polio is about to be. All that is needed is childhood vaccination of everyone—yet the poor child who has already contracted it in the uterus of an unvaccinated, infected mother, while born immune to rubella for life, may well be deaf or worse for life as well. Here are a few simple facts about rubella:

- •Do not ever get vaccinated against rubella during pregnancy.

- •Rubella is most dangerous in early pregnancy as far as fetal deformities are concerned. Thus, if the disease is contracted in the first three or four months, abortion, if morally acceptable, is the treatment of choice.

- •Your children can be vaccinated while you are pregnant.

- •Do not get pregnant 60 days subsequent to your vaccination.

- •If you have never been vaccinated or are not immune (your obstetrician can tell you), then get vaccinated before you leave the hospital after delivery. You will not infect your newborn, even if you breast-feed, and you are not likely to get pregnant for the next two months. We still don't know whether revaccination is necessary.

- •If you have neglected your children's vaccination program, make sure your daughters are tested and, if necessary, vaccinated at the time they go for their premarital blood test. This, incidentally, is already the law in at least one state.

Report to your doctor if you have fever, runny eyes, sore throat, swollen glands, and a rash. It might be one of the other TORCH disorders—by now I am sure you are so spooked you will report anything—but the other disorders are equally or more damaging. So it may pay to be a little spooked.

Cytomegalovirus (CMV)

CMV is but another member of the herpes virus family, and it resides only in humans. It can be transmitted by any number of human fluids, including saliva, tears, urine, blood, semen, cervical secretions, and even breast milk. High-risk environments for contagion include day-care centers, newborn nurseries, mental institutions, renal-dialysis centers, and hospital areas treating immuno-compromised individuals. It can be transmitted across the placenta by infected mothers and may have no fetal effects at all. Rarely, it may produce a number of congenital problems. Thus, although up to 2 percent of all infants may be born with CMV, less than 1 in 20,000 are seriously damaged.

CMV may generate no symptoms when contracted, or it may cause mild flu-like complaints. Routine prenatal testing is not usually done for this agent because tests are not uniformly reliable. There is no vaccine at present and no treatment. Women exposed to CMV by their work environment are sometimes screened, although, again, screening is very complex and not always reliable.

Herpes Virus II (HSVII)

This very prevalent, sexually transmitted virus rarely produces systemic symptoms, but the distribution and character of the shallow, painful ulcers are almost enough to establish a diagnosis. A smear and culture of any open ulcer can be absolutely diagnostic. Herpes lesions are generally found around the vaginal and rectal entrance or inside the vagina, and they may also be found orally, like the common "cold sores" (HSVI). Because of our sexual lifestyles, both HSV I and II may be found orally or genitally, although most genital lesions are HSVII.

Genital HSVII infections seriously complicate the delivery process. Should an infant be delivered vaginally while the HSVII virus is being actively shed in that area, it can sustain massive damage or death. Thus, under those circumstances, cesarean section is the treatment of choice. Some women who have had active HSV genital infections that are inactive at delivery time, or who have had a prophylactic treatment with appropriate acyclovir within a few weeks of delivery, may be considered candidates for a vaginal delivery. This is another very complex area where you must rely upon advice provided by your obstetrician.

The treatment of HPV I or II is, as noted, acyclovir—an antiviral agent that is very effective and can be taken orally for about ten days. Again, your obstetrician knows the dosage range and can tell you about the safety of this medication.

Incidentally, acyclovir also comes as a cream that provides local care for HSVI oral cold sores.

Other Infectious Disorders

Closing the door on the miserable TORCH family still leaves us with other infectious disorders to consider—infections that can have an impact on pregnancy and on our lives. Of all these disorders, none can equal the disastrous impact of AIDS.

Human Immune-deficiency Virus (HIV) and Acquired Immune Deficiency Syndrome (AIDS)

Acquired immune deficiency syndrome (AIDS) is a systemic disease caused by the human immune-deficiency virus (HIV). The HIV incubation period may be as long as ten years and cause few, if any, symptoms! More than 500,000 Americans are afflicted with AIDS, and many, many more carry the HIV precursor. It is now the third-leading cause of death among women 25–44 years of age.

There is practically no risk of contracting the disorder by casual contact. Transmission is almost always through sexual intercourse or by drug injecting—although a very small and very unfortunate number of cases have occurred among health care workers by accidental needle sticks and the like. The fastest-growing category of AIDS cases is women who acquire the disease through heterosexual intercourse. Moreover, since the number of asymptomatic women with HIV is ten times greater than those with full-blown AIDS, it is clear that the disease will continue to spread rapidly. AIDS is gradually making inroads into all levels and age groups, and thus any casual sexual contact can no longer be considered casual. Safe sex is a long-term, mutually monogamous relationship. We can take it or we can leave it.

The symptoms of early AIDS are many, varied, and difficult to classify. If I say that fatigue, weight loss, and flu-like complaints represent a characteristic onset, then every little sniffle will have us convinced that AIDS is at the doorstep. However, if you have any significant reason to suspect or fear AIDS, get to your doctor.

Unrecognized AIDS in women has far-reaching consequences. It not only affects her and her sexual contacts but perhaps any future offspring. The transmission of AIDS to unborn children may be as high as 30 percent and is already the fifth-leading cause of death of children aged 1–4! AIDS progresses rapidly in children—the average time from diagnosis to death is 14 months. Most infants born of infected mothers will carry their mother's HIV antibodies (even if they don't have AIDS) for as long as 15 months after delivery, and this makes the diagnosis of AIDS in these youngsters much more difficult. If AIDS does not exist, these antibodies disappear without doing any harm. Fortunately, there now exists a combination drug program that may protect the unborn child against maternal AIDS transfer.

The management of an AIDS pregnancy is very complex. Frequent testing for AIDS' destructive blood activity is necessary as well as observation for the development of complicating infections such as tuberculosis and other serious lung disorders. These risks seem to multiply at this time: pregnancy has a hastening effect on AIDS progression. Medical agents used to treat AIDS now must be directed at both mother and unborn child. While cesarean section is not necessarily indicated for delivery, special precautions to minimize vaginal-fetal contact must be observed. Breast-feeding the newborn must be avoided.

Routine prenatal AIDS testing is not yet common in all American communities, although some inner-city clinics report that one woman in 60 of childbearing age is infected with the HIV virus. Routine AIDS prenatal testing has been strongly recommended by most medical and public health leaders and may eventually become federal law—just like the syphilis test we talked about earlier. There are various state and local laws concerning screening, reporting, and disclosure, but there is a compelling need for national standards. This is a difficult goal to achieve in today's world, and for a number of reasons. One of the most significant problems is retaining confidentiality. At one time, what you told your doctor, and whatever tests your doctor performed, remained confidential and sealed in your personal medical history. Not so today. Insurers, hospitals, managed care providers, even the government—all have access to your records, whether you know it or not. Almost anyone with a computer, Internet access, and a little hacking skill can explore your records, my records, or virtually any medical records!

It is a wise decision, however, to be tested by your physician if you have any suspicion whatsoever that you may have this virus. Home testing kits for AIDS are available. They require you to stick your finger for some blood, drop it on a treated paper, and then send it off to a laboratory. The lab will call you with the results after you give the password. Private though that procedure is, a positive test would be of no use to you—or to your passenger—unless you reported it to your physician. And there we are again—in the public domain.

It is also important for us all to recognize that physicians have, along with a duty to protect their patient's privacy, a public duty to protect others from serious health hazards. Often this conflict places them in a treacherous position—like grasping a falling sword!

Lyme Disease

There is a danger lurking in the woods in many American communities each summer that may adversely affect normal pregnancies. It is a deer tick that is no larger than the head of a pin. Its presence, therefore, often goes unnoticed by its host, and the first symptoms of the disease it carries often occur weeks after the tick has departed.

First, a circular series of inflammatory skin lesions are seen at the spot of the original bite; these are often accompanied by general flu-like symptoms. Weeks, months, or years later, systemic inflammatory disorders may appear. These include migratory joint pains as well as neurological and cardiac symptoms. The bacteria causing Lyme disease resembles, but is not related to, syphilis.

During pregnancy, the bacteria responsible for Lyme disease can and does cross the placental barrier. Depending on the stage of pregnancy at which that transfer occurs, there can be a variety of serious fetal defects, or there can be intrauterine fetal loss, premature labor, or a number of growth and mental retardation problems.

The disease, which can be diagnosed by certain blood tests, responds to several antibiotics. Many physicians, suspecting that the disease is present in a particular pregnancy, will treat the patient with antibiotics even before the blood tests become positive.

Avoid gamboling in the woods during June, July, and August, particularly if you live in New York, Connecticut, New Jersey, Wisconsin, Minnesota, Massachusetts, Pennsylvania, California, Rhode Island, Texas, or Arkansas. These states are where the tick's presence has been most widely documented.

Fifth Disease

This mild infectious disorder, also known as "slapped-face" syndrome, did not get its name from whiskey. It just happened to be the fifth disease recognized and identified among a group of somewhat similar rash-producing ailments: measles, German measles, chicken pox, and roseola. Medically called erythema infectiosum, this disorder is caused by the human parvovirus B19.

The illness usually runs a mild course with low-grade fever, malaise, and a rash that generally starts on the face and rapidly spreads to the rest of the body. Sometimes there is arthritis-like pain in the wrists, hands, and knees. The incubation period is four to twelve days, and the illness lasts from five to ten days. Schools and day-care centers form a large reservoir for fifth disease.

Rarely, very serious problems may develop when pregnant women contract this disorder. Although population-based studies suggest that up to 4 percent of pregnant women develop B19 while pregnant, less than 2 percent of those infants will be affected. Fetal death in the first and second trimester has been shown to follow fifth disease, as has fetal hydrops (severe anemia along with massive body fluid collections) in the third trimester. Again, these drastic complications are, fortunately, very rare. B19 is not a teratogenic infection.

Fifth disease represents an occupational risk for pregnant women who work in day-care centers or in schools, particularly in the spring months. Tests are available to determine whether you are immune to this disorder, and some suggest that such testing might soon be included in routine prenatal assessment. Blood tests are also available to test for its development during pregnancy. If you do get fifth disease at this time, ultrasound and maternal serum alpha-fetoprotein (MSAFP) (see page 284) tests are useful in assessing the possibility of fetal damage. Other more complex tests are also available to assess the degree of fetal involvement with B19, and intrauterine fetal therapy at research centers has been initiated but is still considered experimental and of unproven value.

Systemic Maternal Infections

There is no question that fetal health is a reflection of maternal health in ever so many ways. Systemic maternal infections that do not directly attack the unborn can still exact a toll upon its well-being. So it is that acute and chronic infections of the lungs, kidneys, or other organ systems must be evaluated and, when possible, controlled. These important health components will all be evaluated as we move on.

So—you may now consider yourself in the flow as far as infectious disorders are concerned, and you are probably happy to get on out. Unfortunately, for the moment anyway, things aren't going to get much brighter!

Teratogens

We have already talked in broad terms in chapter 1 about the risks of medications and drugs during pregnancy. Total avoidance of drugs during pregnancy is a defensible but hardly realistic position. Sometimes it is absolutely necessary to use some therapeutic agent during pregnancy, but most often it is not. Remember these key points:

- About 90 percent of pregnant women take some medication other than their vitamins.

- Some 10 percent take 10 to 19 other drugs, and 6 percent actually take more than 20. That's a fact!

- Forty percent of these medicines are taken in the first trimester.

- At the end of one year, 5 percent of all newborns have demonstrated developmental abnormalities that are probably drug-related. This figure, however, includes the abuse of the drug alcohol and also includes many minor abnormalities.

- Some medications are known to accumulate in the baby's circulation, and sometimes the accumulation is much in excess of that in the mother's.

The most dangerous agents ingested during pregnancy are called **teratogens**. Teratogens produce physical deformities in the fetus. Others, called **clastogens**, can, in a toxic way, damage the fetus without necessarily making visible or detectable structural alterations. Here is a list of *some* of the major identifiable medications and drugs, both prescription and over-the-counter, that have known destructive fetal effects.

Prescription Drugs

Teratogens

thalidomide (formerly a sedative available in other countries only, but now available here to manage leprosy and certain skin and neurological, nonobstetrical health problems)

Dilantin (a cerebral relaxant)

warfarin (an anticoagulant)

folic acid antagonist (generally present in anticancer drugs)

androgens and progestins (hormones)

diethylstilbestrol (DES, an estrogen-like hormone)

mercury (present in some medications)

Accutane (used to treat acne)

Suspected Teratogens

 lithium (a psychiatric drug)

 benzodiazepines (tranquilizers)

 certain oral contraceptives

 amphetamines (stimulants, on the street called "ice," formerly taken
  for weight control)

 cortisone (an anti-inflammatory)

 certain antihistamines

Clastogens

 propranolol (an antihypertensive drug)

 thiazides (diuretic drugs)

 chloramphenicol (an antibiotic)

 tetracyclines (antibiotics)

 meprobamate (a tranquilizer)

 reserpine (antihypertensive)

 erythromycin (an antibiotic)

 streptomycin (an antibiotic)

Over-the-Counter Drugs

Proven Human Teratogens

 ethyl alcohol

Suspected Human Teratogens

 none

Clastogens

 aspirin

 tobacco

 caffeine

certain antihistamines

vitamins A, D, and K in excess

Under-the-Counter Drugs

Clastogens

every one of them, from acid to grass

Common Medications That Are Probably Safe

penicillin and certain derivatives

acetaminophen

mild narcotics, such as codeine taken *occasionally* for pain

These lists are not complete, but they are close to being so. Nonetheless, in the over-the-counter field alone, there are up to a half-million products available, and it is difficult if not impossible to keep up with all of them. Prescription drugs are classified from A to X, as we have seen earlier. Class A, of which there are very few, are considered safe during pregnancy. Most are listed in class C—pregnancy effects unknown. From class D on, the medications are not to be given during pregnancy except for an extremely compelling indication.

The High-Risk Pregnancy

In the beginning of the book, I said that pregnancy itself is not a disease. But in each succeeding chapter, I open another can of pregnant worms and provide you with something else to worry about! I tell you, for instance, that the chance for a certain complication is 12 percent, and for the next one 8 percent, for the next 20 percent, and so on—when you add it all up for yourself, you find there is a 150 percent chance that something terrible is going to get you or your baby or both of you before it's all over! And so your worrying simply compounds as you await the onset of one of these dreaded maladies that I have thrown out at you!

Well, be of good cheer. Sit down and take one of my favorite mood-altering medications—a chocolate brownie—and then think about it all. Ninety-nine percent of what really goes on is good news. But no one would read the book if I didn't report the bad news along with the good. After all, who would want a book that just said you get pregnant, have a few throw-ups and later on some heartburn and fidget-foot, and then go off somewhere and have a baby?

All the preceding information simply serves to grease my bridgehead leading you on to the subject of high-risk obstetrics—pregnancies that have a greater risk of adverse outcome for mother, child, or both. All obstetricians can and do manage these problems, but in many tertiary care centers (see Regionalized Care in the glossary) they are dealt with by perinatologists—specialists in maternal-fetal medicine who concentrate their efforts on high-obstetrical-risk situations (see Management below).

Who actually is at risk? Well, very young and very old expectant mothers, those with advanced infertility problems, diabetics, hypertensives, cardiacs, the obese, those with renal disease, those whose pregnancy is complicated by AIDS, and others. There are, of course, many categories of problems that constitute high risk, and indeed, a normal pregnancy can suddenly become a high-risk problem when, for instance, hypertension of pregnancy imposes itself (see pages 161–164), or upon the discovery of a very abnormal placental location—placenta previa, for instance (see page 51)—a very large (macrosomic) infant, and so on. Finally, certain areas of high-risk obstetrics are at the cutting edge of our knowledge; that is, some types of pregnancy have occurred only rarely—if ever—before. Examples would be pregnancy following coronary artery bypass surgery or following an organ transplant—even a heart transplant. Such cases are beginning to appear before us for obstetrical care!

Certain of these high-risk situations will be dealt with separately and in more detail. These include diabetes, hypertension of pregnancy, pregnancy in older women and very young women, and so on. It will be impossible, however, to detail the management of every one of the disorders that can complicate pregnancy and elevate it to high-risk.

What we must know in order to deal with a complicated pregnancy is the effect of the disorder on pregnancy and the effect of pregnancy on the disorder. Armed with this information, doctors adapt the pregnancy management to that risk problem. Of course, the outcome is not always what we want or hope for. The safety of expectant mothers, as you already know, is very secure; the pregnancy itself, however, may be touch-and-go in many instances. Remember that many high-risk pregnancies involve mothers who in the past could never have conceived or carried a pregnancy under any circumstances.

Management

Each high-risk pregnancy, then, is managed individually. Those at high risk are seen by their doctors more frequently during pregnancy, and special tests and procedures are called for at varying time intervals. Perhaps an example would make the idea of a management program a little clearer.

Suppose, for instance, we are dealing with a pregnancy in which the expectant mother is burdened with chronic hypertension to a moderately severe degree. In the initial visit, there is a complete evaluation of her cardiovascular capacity, its functional reserve, and her kidney reserve and function. Special dietary, weight, and exercise instructions are given, along with signs to watch for that might indicate impending trouble. The physician treating her hypertension is consulted about her medications and other health matters. The pregnancy is followed very closely, and even if all is going well, beginning at around the 28th week visits to the doctor are scheduled for every two weeks, or perhaps even every week. Her doctor is looking for evidence of increasing hypertension or for the addition of hypertension of pregnancy to the existing problem; for evidence of potential heart failure or kidney failure; and finally, but of equal importance, for evidence of fetal health and well-being. Specific maternal medications may have to be monitored and new ones introduced. On the infant's behalf, the doctor is looking for evidence of intrauterine growth retardation (IUGR) (see pages 160–161) or for placental failure. The nonstress test, the stress test, ultrasound monitoring, and the biophysical profile—all will closely monitor the progress of the pregnancy (see the appendix).

As full term approaches, evidence of fetal maturity will be sought as well as any further evidence of fetal distress. At the most opportune time for both mother and child, delivery will be undertaken by the method calculated to cause the least trauma to both. Labor and delivery must be very closely monitored, appropriate anesthesia made available, and, if there is evidence of fetal distress, a pediatrician, or perhaps a neonatologist, should be in attendance. In the event that neither a perinatologist nor a neonatologist is available, a general obstetrician, with the patient's medical hypertensive consultant, and a pediatrician would be well qualified to handle this pregnancy, labor, and delivery.

This is but one brief example of high-risk pregnancy management, and it is admittedly abbreviated and incomplete. However, it may serve to give you an idea of some of the problems involved in obstetrical risk management.

Usually following the delivery of a high-risk pregnancy, and particularly if there has been fetal distress, the newborn is transferred to an intensive-care nursery, where the pediatricians and neonatologists watch over the child. Regardless, all our well-planned programs sometimes fail and we have a bad outcome. We are, however, gaining rapidly in preventing fetal loss and improving the quality of life for the little survivor. It is also true, no matter how far we advance, that there will always be new and distant barricades to attack and strike down. You, the undelivered, stand at the old barricade and may fear the crossing. We, for the most part, stand on the other side and have the confidence and the knowledge that we can bring you through. That's our part of the covenant. It is not a question of control versus surrender on your part. We are in a real bind, and a captain is in order. And that's enough philosophy.

Here follows, in some detail, a common high-risk pregnancy situation and its management.

Diabetes and Pregnancy

Before insulin was discovered and became generally available, diabetes and pregnancy were almost incompatible. Diabetic women generally didn't live long enough to conceive, and if they did get pregnant, the combination was uniformly lethal to both mother and baby. Nowadays, thank goodness, pregnant diabetics, with help, can share the same happy and successful outcome as their unburdened peers. With help.

The effects of diabetes on pregnancy can be:

- miscarriage—repeatedly

- prematurity and postmaturity

- stillbirth

- congenital malformations

- large infants (macrosomia)

- immature and sick infants

- hypertension of pregnancy

- and more

The effects of pregnancy on diabetes are:

- Marked changes in insulin requirements. Insulin needs may decrease in early pregnancy but generally increase and fluctuate sharply in later pregnancy.

- Increased incidence of metabolic imbalance and tendency to develop acidosis in, blood and tissue because the body tends to burn fat instead of sugar during metabolic imbalance. When fat is metabolized, it breaks down into fatty acid substances, thereby producing acidosis, with the potential for considerable harm to both mother and fetus. This dangerous metabolic change can develop silently and rapidly, particularly in late pregnancy.

- Increased dietary needs to nourish the developing pregnancy.

As you can see, all these conditions have a profound effect on each other and require delicate and exquisite control. The management of a diabetic pregnancy usually, but not always, involves:

- Early hospital admission, for control and evaluation of the diabetes and the pregnancy and to establish rapport between the physician, the patient, nutritionists, and all others involved in this elaborate process.

- Meticulous control of the diet, which often involves a change in dietary habits and the initiation of frequent, multiple feedings. The principle here is to prevent hyperglycemia (excess blood sugar), which is the most critically damaging effect diabetes can have on pregnancy.

- Insulin adjustment and constant readjustment. Today, with modern blood-monitoring devices, most cooperative diabetics can assess their own blood sugar levels and adjust their diet and insulin dosages accordingly.

- Close monitoring of fetal activity and growth. This involves the use of nonstress and stress testing as well as biophysical profiles and amniocentesis (see the appendix).

- Close observation in late pregnancy for evidence of fetal lung maturity and assessment of optimal delivery time.

- Special management of "neglecters." Diabetic patients who fail to follow instructions and advice create many problems during pregnancy. Such unfortunate mothers require special help and assistance for themselves and their babies.

Gestational diabetes has received increasing attention over the past few years as our knowledge about it grows. Over half of the women who are destined to have overt diabetes later in life will develop glucose intolerance (that is, diabetes) during pregnancy—and therefore gestational diabetes. These women will sustain the same complications of pregnancy as an active diabetic. It is therefore very important that the condition be determined at least by the beginning of the third trimester.

Accordingly, almost all pregnant women should have a glucose challenge test between the 26th and 28th week of pregnancy. In this procedure, a measured amount of sugar (glucose) is given and blood tests follow to see how the sugar is metabolized. If the test is not normal, then a full glucose tolerance test is usually undertaken.

Once the diagnosis of gestational diabetes is confirmed, these mothers and their pregnancies are treated exactly as if they were active diabetics, since their pregnancies are fraught with the same complications and problems that an active diabetic faces.

It is equally important that these women be informed of their risk in future pregnancies and, indeed, in future life. Every effort must be made to control their weight, dietary habits, and lifestyles to delay or avert the onset of insulin-dependent diabetes in later years.

There are many variations and substitutions among the procedures I have described that may alter the treatment that a pregnant diabetic or a gestational diabetic will receive from her physician. Moreover, our knowledge advances faster than the printed word can be printed. Therefore, your physician, who is in tune with these advances, is your source of guidance through this potential—but manageable—quagmire.

Other High-Risk Complications

Here are listed most high-risk medical complications of pregnancy. Would there was space here to detail all of them. Your physician is, again, your ultimate source of information on any of them that might be in your way to a successful ending.

- •Problems in the gastrointestinal system
  malnutrition
  liver problems such as cirrhosis and acute and chronic hepatitis
  intestinal surgery, previous intestinal surgery such as bypass,
      stomach stapling procedures, and large surgical resections for
      tumors
  Crohn's disease (ulcerative colitis)

- •Problems in the renal system
  chronic infections (pyelitis)
  renal damage (nephritis and nephrosis)
  renal transplants
  renal dialysis

- •Problems in the cardiovascular system
  anemias of various types
  heart disease such as congenital or rheumatic heart disorders,
      ischemic heart disease (angina and/or infarction)
  previous heart surgery for congenital or rheumatic heart disease
      or valve replacement, coronary bypass surgery, and other
      more exotic heart procedures, including heart transplant!
  hypertension and stroke

- •Problems in the endocrine system
  diabetes
  thyroid disorders
  pituitary and adrenal gland disorders

• Problems in the pulmonary system
    asthma, emphysema, and pulmonary infections
    previous surgery to lungs (lobectomy or pneumonectomy)

• Problems involving systemic infection
    TORCH Syndrome
    AIDS

• Problems in the central nervous system
    epilepsy
    migraine
    multiple sclerosis
    cerebral palsy

• Cancer
    arrested cancers of various body organs and systems
    active cancer under therapy

These various disorders are but a sampling of the medical problems that may complicate pregnancy. There are others, and they all serve as a great challenge to modern obstetrical management. As you can see, modern medicine, while prolonging and enhancing life, along with modern infertility procedures, is delivering to obstetricians—and to the women with whose care they have been entrusted—a vast array of new problem pregnancies.

Men's Room—Pregnancy 101

Men: Hail! Good news! Now you can share, at least in a small, short-term way, the very personal and fulfilling sensations and feelings of being pregnant—glorious sensations once experienced only by your lucky pregnant mate! What wonders modern science has blessed you with!

So, yes, let's welcome the baby belly (BB)! This amazing breakthrough in medical research has provided some childbirth preparation groups with the opportunity to harness participating fathers into a remarkable device. Weighing at least 30 pounds, the BB straps on in front and reproduces, at least in part, the excess breast and abdominal mass freely provided to pregnant women, thus closely mimicking at least the heavy front part of their load. The BB comes complete with built-in fluid compartments containing lead spheres to mimic fetal movements as the spheres slosh about—except that they are inactive at night, when the little one is often most active. Oh, well, you can't have everything, men. Still, the lucky fathers chosen to wear this device get to slip it on for a 24-hour period or thereabouts.

Those who have reported tell us, of course, that falling on their face (and on their precious lead-laden BB) was the most common mishap of a physical nature to befall them. Also frequently noted were the experiences of trapping the BB in elevator and train doors; driving turned into a miserable and dangerous adventure; a frustrating inability to stand up to a bar; an equally frustrating inability to dress below the waist; when dressed, the inability to find a certain basic and important zipper (or anything else in that general area); and a significant amount of "wetting" while performing a basic function about which they had previously been very proud—sometimes even competitive!

In the long run—which turned out to be a few hours—ties (when worn) and shirts became soiled and, wonder of wonders, backaches developed. The most disturbing reports—clearly not printable here—centered on nighttime problems. It was very clear, though, that a number of basic habits, customs, rights, and learned functions suffered during the hours of darkness!

So now we may have a subset of believers—men who are willing, perhaps for the first time ever, to at least examine some of the problems their partners refer to from time to time during the perfectly normal physiological course of pregnancy.

Even the most ardent wearers of the BB, and even the most caring obstetrician (unless she *herself* has born children), cannot begin to comprehend what it is like to carry a child into this world. Many things, therefore, must be taken on faith and believed. Do it!

To begin with, there are basic physical, hormonal, and emotional alterations of great magnitude—all of which express themselves in some way as pregnancy moves along. For instance, the powerful hormone progesterone, secreted in tremendous quantities during pregnancy, is very necessary for the maintenance of that pregnancy. As a side effect, however, it also raises the mother's body temperature by at least a degree. Later on, temperatures that you and I consider normal become intolerable to her. Bed covers and regular clothing are also intolerable. These discomforts are not minor, and we wouldn't endure them ourselves for very long.

Now that we have laid the groundwork for this little exercise in understanding, let's discuss some of the changes that pregnancy brings to bear upon our loved ones. These changes include the physical, hormonal, emotional, and, probably, sexual modifications that may confront you.

Physical Changes

Normal female posture is markedly altered by the increasing abdominal girth of pregnancy and, to a lesser extent, by breast changes. If you are not lucky enough to have a baby belly, you can get the hang of things by looking at any woman carrying a term baby from the side. Be careful how you look—but look, and then try standing like that. If she doesn't stand like that, she will fall forward and onto a real baby belly! She is downloaded—you are familiar with that term, surely. Anyway, such necessary posture puts a tremendous strain on her sacroiliac joint, and sooner or later it starts to hurt. After her delivery, you must help her tighten up her stretched and loosened abdominal muscles by exercising with her. Otherwise, the backache becomes chronic.

Certain hormones loosen all the body's ligaments, thus making joints unstable and more readily injured. If she were to swing just once like Tiger Woods, she would come apart! Increasing body weight and postural changes only add to this instability. In very rare instances, the pubic bones separate completely and all walking stops.

Mechanical *pressure* from the baby makes her bladder feel full most of the time. Pressure also tends to make her lower extremities swell (edema) so that her legs may feel like stovepipes. Pressure also, along with certain hormones, makes all her veins dilate.

This is just a short outline of the physical and mechanical problems that usually take place. Any of these areas could be explored in depth. For example, because of the pressure on the bladder, involuntary loss of urine is not uncommon, nor are bladder infections. Neither of these events is likely to improve our lady's outlook on life in general and on an unsympathetic companion in particular.

Hormonal Changes

During pregnancy, women are besieged by a number of powerful hormones that are secreted from their ovaries and pituitary gland as well as from the baby's placenta. What side effects do these hormones have?

- In early pregnancy, they cause nausea and fatigue.

- As time goes on, her body heats up—what's cozy for you is a firestorm for her.

- Her breasts become full and tender and begin to leak fluid.

- Later in pregnancy, uterine cramps and leg cramps become a common delight.

- Vasomotor instability (falling out, fainting, swooning, sinking spell) may take place at any time.

- Indigestion, heartburn, gas, and constipation are all possible, owing to hormonal slowdown of the intestinal tract.

- Emotional changes are likely (keep reading).

Emotional Changes

All of the changes above have a significant impact on the emotional life of a pregnant woman. Now add to these things the rational maternal fears: Will I be all right? Will my baby be all right? Will labor hurt? Will he still love me? And want me? Will I ever look good again?. Insomnia, fretful dreams, and nightmares are not the least bit unusual. In fact, I can give you about 50 reasons for insomnia right now! For example, she wakes up after a bad dream sweating hot because you closed the window, her bladder needs attention, and both her legs are cramping, which requires getting up and stamping her feet, which spills some urine and makes the baby do a full Gaynor from her bladder platform, and then the heartburn and fidget-foot starts. Would you like to wake up nights like that? Want to give it a try? Then go run 35 miles, drop in to your favorite Mexican watering hole, load up on tacos and chili—all churning with peppers—wash it all down with a few Texas margaritas, savor it over a couple of pungent cigars, go home, set the alarm for 2:00 A.M., and then crash. Have a good night.

Sexual Changes

Any or all of the above conditions may have a profound effect on a once free-and-easy, unfettered sexual life. Because of local pressure, congestion, and irritation, sexual congress may be unpleasant and uncomfortable for her, particularly in late pregnancy. Moreover, her sexual drive may shift significantly as pregnancy advances. Usually, sex drives diminish and orgasm may be difficult or delayed and may often be accompanied by painful uterine contractions. Sometimes her doctor will restrict sexual activity, particularly if she has a history of premature labor. Sex should also be canceled if there is vaginal bleeding, pain, infection, or ruptured membranes—or most definitely if you have been asked not to.

Listen to her!

Well, men, these are just a few things I wanted to share with you about her situation as her pregnancy unfolds. My list is admittedly incomplete, but you get the idea. Pregnancy, normal though it may often be, is an emotionally and physically tumultuous time, and one that should invite a great deal of compassion, understanding, and love from us all.

More Pregnant Pauses

- In most ancient cultures, the management of the umbilical cord following delivery was handled in a very specific way. In general, the cord was cut after the placenta was completely delivered, but sometimes it was cut beforehand. Usually separation was achieved at some distance from the baby in order that bleeding would not take place. Instead of being cut with a sharp instrument, it was generally chewed or ground apart with stones. Sometimes heat was used to separate it, and sometimes it was simply torn by the hands. It really didn't make much difference, since placental circulation— and therefore circulation through the cord—ceases at the moment of a newborn child's first respiration.

•In ancient Arabic cultures, pieces of raw salt were put into the mother's vagina after she delivered. The purpose of this was to make the vagina shrivel enough so that it would be tight in subsequent sexual encounters. The complications from this practice can be unbelievable. It is still carried out in some nomadic cultures today.

•A new obstetrical phrase has been coined. The phrase "bronco babies" is derived from the rapidly increasing number of babies born in automobiles to mothers trying to get to a hospital. As more and more rural (and urban) doctors stop delivering babies—general practitioners and obstetricians alike—pregnant women are being forced to travel much greater distances to obtain care. In Hawaii, for example, pregnant women must island-hop! The culprit? The risk of being sued (over 70 percent of all obstetricians have been sued at least once) and soaring malpractice costs. In the New England states, as an example, almost half of the obstetricians have stopped delivering babies.

•Children with AIDS constitute the second-fastest-growing group of AIDS patients in the United States today.

•New York State has reinstituted routine testing of newborn infants for syphilis. Congenital syphilis has doubled in that state in recent years. The sudden burst has been attributed to prenatal crack and cocaine use and the exchange of sex for drugs.

•Besides oil, the Gulf War has produced a variety of mysterious medical complaints. Among them, it has been suggested that a number of birth defects sustained by the offspring of American soldiers are directly related to certain exposures during that struggle. A study of some 34,000 such children failed to confirm any relationship.

•Most glucose tolerance tests involve two unpleasant components—a nauseating sugar-cola drink and needle sticks. The cola drink may soon be history. Some thoughtful investigators demonstrated that 18 jelly beans work just as well as the miserable drink. Thus, we have the President Reagan glucose tolerance test!

Diary

My Fourth Month

Problems_____
_____
_____

Medications_____
_____
_____

Baby moved? When?_____
_____
_____
_____

What's going on in the world?_____
_____
_____
_____

What's going on in my life?_____
_____
_____
_____

My thoughts and feelings_____
_____
_____
_____

Doctor's appointment_____
_____
_____

Questions to ask_____

Five

My Fifth Lunar Month

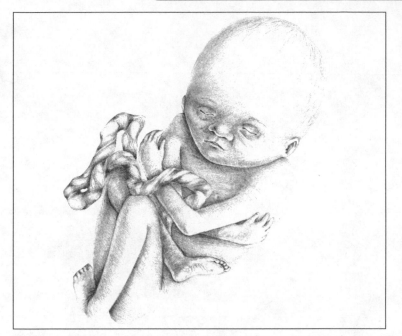

Now in its fifth lunar month, your little passenger weighs about ten ounces (300 grams) and is 7.2 inches (18 centimeters) long. A very soft, downy hair called "lanugo" covers all of its skin, and the skin itself begins to thicken with fat deposits, thus making it less transparent. Some scalp hair may be present.

On ultrasound—as shown here—we can see the facial features, some backbone, and a few dark spots in the chest representing some of the heart chambers. In chapter 8, you will see a cone-down view of a fetal heart (page 198) showing the four chambers as they normally appear. Any abnormalities in the

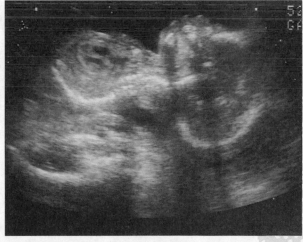

heart chamber appearances or number is of vital importance, since protective and corrective intervention must be taken at birth or—in some centers—even prior to birth by trans-abdominal fetal surgery.

The 16th to the 20th weeks are the fifth lunar month of your pregnancy. During this continuing, rather tranquil time of your pregnancy, your little passenger will break the peaceful spell quite regularly as it practices high dives, broad jumps, and goal-tending, all within the narrow confines of your uterus, and by the end of this month (the 20th week), your uterus, with its athlete, will have risen to your umbilicus. It is very easy now and very reassuring to listen to your baby's heartbeat. You can hear the beat clearly with a stethoscope, and your doctor will produce a heartbeat (from your baby!) that all present can hear using an electronic fetoscope. Of course, an ultrasound taken at this time, for whatever reason, will reveal all.

Immunization During Pregnancy

Sometimes vaccination dilemmas come up in pregnancy. Here is a summary of the known immunization facts.

Four types of immunizing agents are used in the United States:

- **toxoids,** which are chemically altered poisons secreted by bacteria

- **killed bacterial and viral vaccines,** which still retain their ability to produce immunity

- **live virus vaccines,** which have been altered so that they do not cause serious clinical illness but still produce immunity

- **immune globulin preparations,** a protein fraction of human plasma that can induce transient, passive antibody protection in the recipient

Women of childbearing age in this country usually are already immune to measles, mumps, rubella (German measles), tetanus, and diphtheria. Most women born prior to 1957 are considered immune to measles, mumps, and German measles because they most likely were infected with the disease. Those born after 1957 have probably been vaccinated; in fact, most everyone should now have been vaccinated against rubella. Unfortunately, not everyone has. So we are witnessing a resurgence of this dangerous obstetrical infection—an infection that we could eliminate entirely if we would just use what has been given to us. As far as diphtheria and tetanus are concerned, almost everyone has now been vaccinated, although booster doses are required every ten years for diphtheria and tetanus to keep immune levels high.

As a general rule, vaccination with any immunizing agent during pregnancy should be limited to a few very clearly defined situations. Preferably, of course, all routine vaccinations will have been carried out prior to pregnancy. This is not always the case; moreover, some unusual exposures may take place. Each situation must be assessed in terms of the following:

- **Risks of exposure.** Pregnant women should avoid, whenever possible, areas where certain infectious disorders are epidemic or endemic. As an example, avoid travel to areas where the plague or yellow fever exists—and there are areas of the United States where plague now exists. As another example, if you are a teacher, stay home when epidemics of rubella, flu, or chicken pox are active in your school—if you can!

- **Risks from disease.** When a pregnant woman is susceptible and at risk of exposure to an infectious disorder, then the particular mortality and morbidity risks of the disease for her and her fetus must be assessed carefully by her doctors. Some infectious disorders are known to produce greater harm during pregnancy than at other times; rubella is a good example, and we have already seen others.

- **Risks from immunizing agents.** We have to consider further what risk the immunizing agents themselves might have upon the expectant mother, her health, and that of her fetus. Not much is known about the effect of most vaccines on pregnancy. One that has been studied in great detail, however, is rubella and its vaccine; vaccination with this agent is definitely not recommended during pregnancy. On the other hand, diphtheria and tetanus vaccinations are apparently safe at this time.

These factors must all be weighed in making the decision to vaccinate during pregnancy, and all involved need to participate in the decision-making process.

Here is a list of immunizing agents and their status in pregnancy situations.

Toxoids

Tetanus and diphtheria. These vaccinations should have been taken care of during childhood, but since there are no established fetal risks associated with them, vaccination may be undertaken in pregnancy if indicated, and also if indicated, booster shots may be given at this time.

Live Virus Vaccines

Measles and mumps. Routine immunization against these disorders should be avoided during pregnancy. Susceptible women should be vaccinated postpartum.

Poliomyelitis. This vaccine may be given during pregnancy if increased risk of exposure exists. Routine pregnancy vaccination is no longer advised.

Rubella (German measles). This vaccine should not be administered during pregnancy, nor for three months before conception takes place.

Yellow fever. Administer yellow fever vaccine only if exposure to the disease is unavoidable.

Immune Globulins

Hepatitis B. Maternal exposure to this virus may require the protection of immune globulin while pregnant. Should maternal hepatitis B infection actually exist in the mother, appropriate vaccination schedules for the fetus must be followed, as discussed earlier.

Rabies. Post-rabies exposure immune globulin is important at any time to help limit this very dangerous infection.

Tetanus. Post-exposure immune globulin is important at any time during pregnancy. It should be used in conjunction with tetanus toxoid, following all the usual toxoid precautions.

Inactivated Virus Vaccines

Influenza. This vaccine may be given to pregnant women during a severe epidemic, particularly in the presence of significant maternal cardiac or pulmonary disease. State health departments will have all current influenza vaccine recommendations. It is wise to take this very safe (except for people allergic to egg white) vaccine each and every fall. Soon there should be a nasal spray influenza vaccine.

Rabies. Killed rabies virus vaccine should be given to pregnant women only after consultation with health authorities and with the clearest of indications determined on an individual basis.

Hepatitis B. This modern vaccine consists of HBV DNA cultured in certain bacteria! It is therefore one of a new class of vaccines. Although it is a very safe vaccine, it is still a category C agent and thus should be avoided during pregnancy unless there are very compelling reasons for its administration.

Polio. Also available in this inactivated form, this polio vaccine is a category C and should be avoided while pregnant. The whole issue of live versus inactivated polio vaccination is very complex at any time and should be thoroughly discussed with your physician. We can hope that the disease will soon be wiped out and vaccination no longer be needed.

Inactivated Bacterial Vaccines

Cholera, plague, and typhoid. These vaccines should be given only to meet the strictest international travel requirements and with full informed consent of the pregnant traveler.

Pneumococcus. The indications for this vaccine are not altered by pregnancy. It is rarely indicated, and one dose generally confers lifetime immunity.

Meningococcus. Although there are no apparent contraindications for this vaccine during pregnancy, it is indicated only in the most severe and unusual epidemic outbreaks.

In closing this immunization report, you may be interested to learn that a great deal of vaccination research is going on at this moment. At least three large programs are closing in on an HPV vaccine (see chapter 4), and with success, we will have a powerful new weapon to join the Pap smear against cancer of the cervix. Vaccine research to address the HIV disaster is proceeding feverishly, but success still appears to be years away.

As there has been at the crossroads of all medical advances, a reactionary group is squatting at this one. Some people opposed to vaccination allege that it is unsafe, unproved, and not as protective as getting the disease! They should have been around to come with me through the vast children's polio wards not too many years ago. Or they could look through an old family cemetery plot and see how parents were robbed of their little ones by typhoid, diphtheria, scarlet fever, pertussis, smallpox, and on and on. I hope those squatters ban this book!

Traveling

There are some precautions you should consider when traveling by car, by air, or, if internationally, by whatever transportation is at hand—from a stateroom on the *QE2* to the back of a yak!

By Car

If you travel by automobile, try to observe the following guidelines:

•Travel no longer than eight hours a day. Don't travel at all at night.

•Stop frequently. Get out, walk around, stretch your limbs, and test all the reasonable local facilities. The best bathroom facilities appear to be at interstate rest stops and in combination quick food–gas stations. Some rest stops will test your nausea control.

•If your doctor agrees, carry some 50-milligram vitamin B tablets with you in case you become carsick. If you tend to get nauseated, don't read maps, directions, books, or anything. Keep some bland food at hand.

•Always fasten your safety belt, no matter how short the ride. Be sure that the lap belt is below your baby and riding on your thighs and that the shoulder harness gives you at least three inches of freedom in the upper chest area. The benefit to you and baby far outweighs any risks of compression or being trapped in the car. If you are driving the car yourself and are not buckled in, the steering wheel can represent a formidable weapon to both of you. Always buckle up.

•Air bags, as you are aware, are controversial at the moment. If you are not extremely short and are sitting up, the bag should protect you rather than hurt you. Your pregnancy should also be well below the bag's expansion area. At this moment, people are considering whether to disconnect their auto air bags and auto manufacturers are not sure what to do in the future. The last word on the subject will have to come from some source other than this book. One thing is certain: If you are driving, hold the sides of the wheel rather than the top, and wear as little jewelry as possible. You do not want your bejeweled arms and hands shoved into your face by an air bag!

•Be sure you take all your vitamins and other medications along with you.

•Do not make long trips without checking with your doctor first. There are certain times during your pregnancy when it might be unwise for you to be far from home base. Try to avoid travel during the first three months; although traveling itself does not induce a miscarriage, the roadside is no place to have one. Further, traveling during the last month should be avoided because labor may be imminent, and besides, the rest stops are probably not close enough together anymore!

There is nothing worse than long-distance automobile traveling when you are low on gas, high on bladder pressure, tired, hungry, and thirsty, and it is often difficult to find a place to stop that offers all the facilities you need. The National Association of Truck Stop Operators will send you, at a nominal charge, the names of some 500 all-day, all-night auto-truck stops in the United States. These facilities are noted for gas and oil and bathrooms, but they also offer places to sleep, laundries, barbershops, post offices, banks, shopping centers, and the like. Such information might be of real value to you on a long trip. Write to this association at P.O. Box 1285, Alexandria, VA 22313, or call them at (703) 549–2100.

Unless there is something very abnormal with your pregnancy, you may travel within a 30–40-mile radius of home at any time—as long as you buckle up and buckle the kids up in the backseat. It would help to have a cellular phone with you. They are getting more reasonable in price and more powerful.

By Air

Commercial airlines offer the safest way to get about. Air travel is certainly safer (and sometimes faster) than ground travel. There are as yet no airway gridlocks—but some airports are working on it! Smoking—once a great airline hazard—has just about disappeared from commercial carriers in the United States and in international carriers flying to and from the United States. The same cannot be said for carriers in certain other countries. Here are some other points:

- Most American airlines will not allow travel by pregnant women after 36 weeks, and most foreign airlines after 35 weeks. Some require a note from your doctor confirming your due date.

- The radiation involved in airport security devices is not harmful to pregnant women.

- Modern pressurized cabins compare to the altitude found between Denver (5,000 feet) and Crested Butte (8,000 feet), Colorado. These pressures are generally safe for fetal oxygenation but may prove a hazard for anemic pregnant women who live at low altitudes.

- The average humidity level in a commercial aircraft is around 8 percent. Pregnant women lose water rapidly, as you already know. It is therefore important to keep yourself well hydrated on long flights—with water, not alcohol!

- Clotting (thrombosis) in the deep leg veins is a slightly increased hazard during pregnancy. It is a good idea to move around (in a smooth flight) as much as you can. Your bladder will help you in this chore. If weather chains you to your seat, at least keep your legs moving and their muscles contracting.

- Don't eat gas-producing foods before or during your flight. The gas produced will expand in your intestines and cause discomfort during flight.

- Carry your medications with you—not in checked baggage.

- For more information on air travel, write to the Airtransport Association of America, 1709 New York Ave., N.W., Washington, D.C. 20006.

International Travel

If you plan to travel outside the United States, particularly in a foreign country where there may be a language barrier, the International Association for Medical Assistance to Travelers can give you a list of English-speaking physicians almost anywhere in the world. If you wish more information about this society or want its catalog, write to International Association for Medical Assistance to Travelers, 417 Center St., Lewiston, NY 14092.

On a long trip, jet lag increases your fatigue, so be sure to take it easy for the first 24–48 hours after your arrival. This fatigue is even more evident if you are flying to a place of higher altitude than your home. Mountain sickness is a very common complaint among air travelers who fly from sea-level homes to an elevated destination and who do not move around carefully for a day or so. This happens to us flatlanders who fly off to ski—and it is particularly ominous for pregnant flatlanders. Mountain sickness resembles pneumonia, but the treatment is the exact opposite. So start off slowly. Give yourself a day or two to get acclimatized.

Vaccination requirements vary from country to country. You may find the information you need either from your travel agent or from the Centers for Disease Control (CDC) in Atlanta. Call the International Traveler's Information Hotline at (404) 332–4559; for selected information, call (404) 332–4555. Incidentally, most vaccination rules in foreign countries are to protect them—not you!

If you are susceptible to diarrhea and are traveling abroad, remember that roughly half the Americans visiting foreign countries end up with "turista"—some of it caused by relatively harmless E. coli bacterial infestations, but some of it brought on by more serious salmonella and other virulent organisms. Remember, drink bottled water and avoid iced drinks and uncooked or lightly cooked foods. Peel all fruits (although you can't peel raspberries!), and wash and peel all vegetables.

As you all know, we have our own E. coli at home. Some recent coli types—so far found mainly in hamburger meat—are even becoming very dangerous. We are more likely to be immune to, or less sensitive to, our own American *E. coli* bacteria than to the different strains in other countries, where food inspections may be as stringent as our own—or more so. It is just that we are more sensitive to foreign strains. As a matter of fact, there are even regional *E. coli* strains in our own country. Thus, easterners may luck into a different strain when visiting in San Francisco and so leave more than their hearts behind.

As a matter of fact, Americans no longer have to leave the United States to get "turista." So much of our foodstuffs are now imported that the disorder is being brought right into our kitchens. Thus, you read about strawberries from Mexico and raspberries from Guatemala introducing widespread gastrointestinal disease outbreaks in America. The problem is further compounded by the widespread American food distribution networks, through which contaminated food occasionally slips, striking various locations nationwide.

These widespread outbreaks have prompted investigations by the CDC both here and abroad and prompted federal legislation to try to halt the spread of foodborne illness.

The over-the-counter drugs Pepto-Bismol and Imodium A-D are helpful in controlling moderate diarrhea. Imodium A-D has no teratogenic effects on laboratory animals but has not been studied in humans. Trimethoprim-sulfamethoxazole (Bactrim) has recently been approved by the FDA for the management of traveler's diarrhea. Bactrim is a category C drug, so it must be used with caution. You might consider taking all these medications abroad with you, since the benefits may vastly outweigh the risks in a difficult, remote setting. Diarrhea that persists or is accompanied by fever, dehydration, or bloody bowel movements needs immediate medical attention. Powdered Gatorade, which you might also want to take along, can be dissolved in pure water or soda water and will help maintain fluid and electrolyte balance.

One final point about international travel to keep in mind: Vehicular injuries are *the* major cause of death among American travelers abroad. Seat belts and safe drivers are often hard to come by. Add to that narrow roads, absence of speed limits, and, in some countries, reversal of our driving patterns, and you can see why the risks are so great. Your best bet? Rent a sturdy wagon with seat belts, drive yourselves, practice left-side driving and managing roundabouts, and avoid the autobahn!

Trauma and Accidents

At least one in every twelve pregnant women sustains some form of trauma, and sad to say, trauma and violence are the second-leading cause of death among all women of reproductive age—preceded only by AIDS! In some parts of our country, the "trauma" of homicide is the number-one cause of maternal death. What a tragic statistic.

A major traumatic source of pregnancy injuries is the roadway.

Automobile Accidents

Even in a minor accident, you may not remember very much about the moment of impact, and so you may not be certain whether you received an abdominal blow. If you are able to, check at once by feeling around your tummy to see whether there is any area of tenderness. Also check for bruising. As soon as you have a chance, try to determine whether there has been any change in your vaginal secretion; look in particular for the presence of blood or water. If there is the least doubt in your mind, go to a hospital and get examined, and be sure to ask for a fetal heart check. You may want to repeat the monitor check the next day in your doctor's office. Unless it is unavoidable, don't take any medication for pain or for anything unless your obstetrician or doctor orders it.

In a major accident, if you are conscious, tell someone that you are pregnant, how far along you are in the pregnancy, what your blood type happens to be, and the name of your doctor.

Home Falls

Landing on your back or your side, if you fall, generally cushions the blow for the baby. But if the fall is severe and sudden, it may indirectly produce damage to the baby. So if you fall, you must watch for abdominal pain, vaginal bleeding or fluid, and, if the baby has already been moving, any change in the amount of activity. If you fall on or get hit on your abdomen, again, check for pain or bleeding and the amount of baby activity. If you are in doubt, call your doctor or go to a hospital and have them listen with the fetal heart monitor.

Sometimes after you have had a spill or a fright of some sort, your baby becomes very active. After all, baby is in there in the dark, standing on its head, unable to see or hear what's going on. To add even more fetal insult, your injury releases a flood of adrenaline into your system— adrenaline that quickly flows into your baby's circulation. No wonder it jumps around when you have a violent reaction to something!

Fall-proof your home as much as possible. Remove throw rugs, light passageways, slip-proof tubs and showers, and wear safe shoes. In public, don't be embarrassed to use handicapped runways.

Thermal Burns, Electric Shock, and Lightning

Severe thermal burns usually do not affect the baby. Electric shocks can, depending upon where the current comes in and where it goes out.

Again, look for these three cardinal signs: pain, vaginal bleeding, and loss of the sensation of baby movement. Get a fetal monitor check if necessary. Let your doctor know.

Even supposing we find out the very worst—that your baby has been lost even though you're okay—there is nothing that can now be done to change what has happened. It has to be somehow borne and accepted. Moreover, it is important to know. An infant no longer alive cannot be left inside very long because of the harmful effects it may have upon the mother.

On the brighter side, what a blessing it is after such injury to find out that your baby is alive and fine—and that's almost always the case!

Abuse

This subject has not been covered in previous editions of this book because not enough was known about it that could be considered factual. Now, sadly, there is an abundance of statistics about this terrible activity—which is either growing rapidly or being reported more thoroughly. Or both.

Studies reveal that abuse may take place in 17 percent of all pregnancies! Moreover, women abused at this time suffered a greater constellation of symptoms than their abused nonpregnant sisters. Whereas accident victims tend to sustain peripheral body injuries, abused pregnant women are more likely to sustain multiple injuries of the face, neck, breasts, and abdomen. There is a wealth of further frightening statistics available to embarrass and alarm us—but enough is enough. This problem exists.

More and more physicians are being trained to look for and to understand abusive relationships among their patients. We now realize that the most useless and abrasive question that we can ask is, "Why don't you just leave?" Clearly it is not that simple—not by a long shot. Leaving is a drawn-out and difficult problem with many setbacks and slipbacks.

If your physician has been unable to elicit that information or to discover abusive signs, it is still important that she or he be made aware of the situation. Even if direct abdominal blows do not damage the baby or start labor, the abusive situation itself may induce preterm labor, chorioamnionitis (infection within the amniotic fluid), and other obstetrical problems of significant magnitude.

Physical abuse during pregnancy crosses all economic and social barriers and is probably a by-product of our increasingly violent society. That is an explanation—not a defense. There is no defense.

Vaginal Bleeding

Vaginal bleeding anytime during pregnancy must be considered an abnormal sign (although it may not be) and should be reported to your doctor immediately. Often it signifies no great danger, but its importance should be evaluated by your doctor and no one else. As we have seen, bleeding in early pregnancy is a common sign of a threatened or impending miscarriage. Now that you are further along, there are many other sources of vaginal bleeding, among them such relatively benign conditions as infections of the vagina or the cervix or minor varicose veins in this area. Occasionally a small amount of spotting may be noted after sexual relations, owing to irritation of the vagina and the cervix, but still, let your doctor know.

The most dangerous type of bleeding that can occur now is from the site of the placenta. Such bleeding usually signifies that part of the placenta has separated from the uterine wall; it may or may not be accompanied by pain. Whatever the other symptoms, you should call your doctor at once whenever significant vaginal bleeding appears.

Sometimes, as full term approaches, labor is initiated by the discharge of a plug of mucus from the cervix, which many times is stained with blood. This discharge is called "show" and is not a cause for worry. Labor may start within a few moments after the appearance of show, but it may not begin for several hours or even days. There is no need to call your doctor when show appears unless it is accompanied by other signs of labor, such as regular cramps, or unless the membranes rupture. These signs are all explored further along in your book.

Twins and More

Once you have found out for sure that you are pregnant, know when to expect delivery, and are aware that the sex can now be determined with reasonable accuracy and simplicity using modern ultrasound, your next question may well be, "Could I be carrying twins? Or triplets? Or . . . more?"

Well, you certainly could, particularly if you are over 30 and have several children already, if twinning is in your family history, and if your uterus has some abnormal shape. Your chances under such a combination of circumstances would be about 1 in 20. The chances are much greater if you have been taking fertility drugs or if you are involved in a fertility program.

Ordinarily, you have about a 1 in 80 chance (slightly greater if you are black) of twinning, about 1 in 80×80 (6,400) of having triplets, 1 in $80 \times 80 \times 80$ (512,000) for quadruplets, and so on. These are rough projections, and many things can affect them. As mentioned, recent medical advances in the management of infertility have definitely altered this mathematical formulation. The techniques employed can induce multiple ovulation as well as seed the uterus with a multiple number of fertilized embryos. As an example of these advances, in 1997 an American couple produced seven live infants (septuplets), at least partly as a result of a fertility program with which they were involved.

The rate of regular twinning varies throughout the world from very high—40 per 1,000 in Nigeria—to a low of .4 per 1,000 in the Orient. The rate of identical twinning is constant worldwide; it is the rate of fraternal twinning that alters these figures.

Here are some more facts about multiple pregnancies.

- **Monozygotic** twins are identical. They come from the initial split of one egg. Inheritance, maternal age, and the number of previous children have no influence on identical twinning, and as noted, the rate is universally constant.

- **Dizygotic** (two-egg), or fraternal twins, are definitely more common in older women with previous children and a family history of twins. Incidentally, twins do not skip a generation.

- **Superfetation** produces twins in an unusual way. It is based upon the development of a second fertilized egg within a uterus that already contains a developing pregnancy from a previous cycle. Thus, these twins are of different ages and present us with unusual problems. **Superfecundation,** once thought to be even more unusual, results from two or more eggs that ovulated in the same cycle being fertilized by sperm from two different episodes of intercourse, either by the same or a different partner. Recent observations, however, confirm that this is not so unusual an event.

- **Malformations** of the uterus—a double uterus, for instance—seem to predispose a pregnancy toward twins.

- How to tell if twins are identical or fraternal:
    If the sexes are different, they are obviously fraternal.
    If the twins are in one amniotic sac, they are identical.
    If the amniotic sacs are separated by four layers (a microscopic determination), the twins are fraternal; if by only two layers, they are identical.
    One placenta means identical twins, but two placentas—or even conjoined placentas—can be found in either type of twin.
    In difficult cases, extensive blood typing and DNA analysis will absolutely confirm the relationship.

- Triplets and quadruplets may come from one egg, but this is unusual. More often several eggs are involved. The famous Dionne quintuplets, for instance, came from three eggs.

Multiple births generally happen prematurely—three weeks early for twins, on the average—and of course these babies are smaller, not only because they are born early but because there was less room inside and less food to go around. Twins weigh about the same as a singleton up until about the 20th week of gestation and thereafter gain at a consistently slower rate. Twins born in a first pregnancy are likely to be smaller than those in a later pregnancy. Identical twins tend to be smaller and to weigh about the same. They also, unfortunately, have a slightly greater tendency to have more deformities because the single egg may not have split evenly or completely. The difference in weight may be much greater in fraternal twins, and in fact, if they are the result of superfetation, there may be a considerable difference. Also, one rascal may even steal nourishment from the placenta of its wombmate, resulting in a tremendous weight difference.

Plural pregnancies and deliveries are subject to many more complications, such as anemia, hydramnios (excess amniotic fluid), hypertension of pregnancy, edema, difficult and premature labor, and delivery with abnormal presentation.

Twins are generally but not always diagnosed before delivery. The doctor becomes suspicious when there is rapid weight gain and a rapid increase in uterus size, with many small parts to feel. Ultrasound examination reveals with almost 100 percent accuracy whether twins are present. Incidentally, modern ultrasound can also tell us, with significant accuracy, when labor may be very early in multiple pregnancies because it will clearly demonstrate the length of the cervical canal. With a very long canal, labor is usually far off.

Occasionally twins are incorrectly diagnosed because what appears to be a second fetal sac in early pregnancy may be either a false sac or a second embryo that reabsorbs (see the appendix). Thus, it may be that many pregnancies start out as twins and end up as singletons; only further ultrasound research will establish this possibility. Ultrasound occasionally overlooks one baby of triplets or quadruplets, but it is, by and large, exceedingly accurate in making the determinations I have outlined.

With the advent of multiple pregnancy states that involve many infants, **fetal reduction** has become an established procedure. As an example, let us say that seven fetuses are clearly identified by ultrasound. Statistics and actual results have made it clear that the chances of any of them surviving are minimal. Accordingly, it is acceptable to destroy several of these fetuses to increase the survival chances of those remaining. This can be accomplished with little risk to the mother or to the remaining infants. Sometimes an abnormal-appearing fetus or a smaller fetus is sacrificed; sometimes it is just chance or proximity to the abdominal wall that determines which one or ones are selected for reduction by transabdominal procedures. Such procedures clearly present a moral dilemma that not all of us can readily resolve—despite the logic that drives it on. The American couple mentioned earlier chose to forgo fetal reduction. However, it is now an accepted practice.

If you are expecting more than one child, it is important that you spend a fair part of the last third of your pregnancy at rest. You should be up only to take care of basic functions. You may be plagued by boredom, insomnia, swelling, pressure, and thoughts about how to improve your bedroom ceiling, but bed rest is essential. Bed rest apparently does not necessarily hold back the onset of premature labor, but it helps prevent hypertension of pregnancy, a common complication with twins, and it does increase fetal nourishment and therefore fetal weight at the time of birth. This is all very important. While you are in bed, keep body muscle toned as much as you can by isometric exercise, but *do not bear down.* Management of labor and delivery of multiple births should generally be in a class II or III obstetrical unit (see the discussion of perinatal centers in the appendix). It can become a very complicated procedure, and the incidence of cesarean section is somewhat greater for twin deliveries than for singletons.

For more information about multiple births, write to the Triplet Connection, 2618 Lucille Ave., Stockton, CA 95209 (209–474–0885), or the National Organization of Mothers of Twins Clubs, Inc., 12404 Princess Jeanne, N.E., Albuquerque, NM 87112 (505–275–0955).

Backache and Posture

Perhaps one of the most significant differences between people and animals is our ability to walk erect, but alas, our erect posture has led to that exclusively human disorder: the aching sacroiliac. The sacroiliac joint is your means of connecting two very important body parts to each other: your top to your bottom. Thus, this area is a common source of considerable discomfort when abused or damaged. It is, after all, a pivot point that must turn and bend hundreds of times each day.

There are many ways of stressing, straining, and, eventually, damaging the lower back. Being overweight, lifting improperly, poor posture, diseases and injuries—all are contributors. Pregnancy is another one of them. Your growing baby acts like a weight and pulls you forward. To compensate for this, you lean further back and increase the strain and the shearing effect on your sacroiliac area. If your unindicted co-conspirator can't understand how this happens, ask him to hang his bowling ball on his belt buckle for a few days!

After delivery, backache sometimes persists for a long time and may eventually develop into a chronic low-back strain unless corrective postural exercises are done regularly or some supportive mechanism is worn. Various plans and devices can help combat the chronic sacroiliac strain:

- In early pregnancy, try wearing an ordinary stretch **girdle** until it is no longer comfortable. Then a good maternity shop can supply you with a lightweight girdle that will give you excellent support for the remaining months of pregnancy (see page 72). Although these girdles are not the massive binders of old, they actually are pretty restrictive and, in the summertime, very hot. Unless your back is extremely painful, it's probably better to avoid any kind of girdle, since these devices tend to do the work your muscles should be doing in the first place.

- Do **postural exercises.** Instruction booklets provided by the American College of Obstetricians and Gynecologists are generally available at your doctor's office.

- During periods of rest and upon retiring at night, **sleep on your side.** Curl up as much as you can and put a pillow between your legs. This helps relieve the sacroiliac strain and discomfort.

- If it's absolutely necessary, take **medicine** that reduces the spasm and inflammation around the sacroiliac joint, but only under your doctor's supervision.

- After delivery, **exercise** more diligently. Vigorous postural exercises are preferable to wearing a girdle. You will find that you are getting plenty of exercise after you arrive home from the birthing center and may not be pleased that your doctor and I are suggesting a few more. Actually, however, most of the work that you do doesn't help your back a bit; it probably tends to make your strained joints more strained. Your back is going to have to carry you a long way and for a long time—so be kind to it. Do the appropriate exercises.

If you have a really bad back with chronic disability arising from an injury or a disease, it is important that you have an orthopedic consultation. If any back surgery is suggested, it is very wise to get a second opinion from another orthopedist or a neurologist. Back surgery is fraught with problems.

Teeth for Two

Pregnant women are often warned by friends and relatives that their teeth are going to fall out while they are pregnant. "For every child, a tooth" is a folklore saying that has survived from antiquity, and it drives dentists up the wall. Perhaps there is an element of truth in it, but if there is, research has failed to prove it. Calcium deposited in the teeth is ordinarily not available again to the circulation. So no matter how badly calcium is needed elsewhere, even for the bones and teeth of a developing infant, it generally cannot be reabsorbed from an expectant mother's teeth. Enamel is permanent, so that cavities that occur during pregnancy are coincidental to—not caused by—enamel loss. Moreover, if you faithfully take the prenatal vitamins your doctor prescribed, there is only a slight possibility of a calcium deficiency developing during your pregnancy. (Contrary to popular belief, milk may not be a good source of calcium during pregnancy. The calcium in milk is poorly absorbed by pregnant women. See pages 211–212.) If extra calcium is necessary, for any reason, calcium carbonate tablets are a cheap and excellent source of that mineral.

You should see your dentist early in pregnancy to be sure your teeth are in good condition. Any necessary dental work may be done during pregnancy, but gas anesthetics should not be used. You may have any form of local anesthetic your dentist wishes to use—provided you have no allergies to the local medication. Elective extractions should be delayed.

An unusual swelling of the gums is seen during pregnancy. This is almost never due to any vitamin deficiency but to a vascular change in the gums. There is redness and swelling in the gum mucosa, and it often produces bleeding upon slight contact. Hormonal changes induce this gum mucosa effect, and it disappears promptly after pregnancy is over.

Stuffy Nose and Ears

The same congestion of superficial veins that sometimes takes place in the gums is seen frequently in the mucous membranes of the nose and ear canals. Remember the following:

• When swelling occurs in the nasal passages, besides bothersome nasal congestion, nosebleeds may be the result. As a rule, such bleeding doesn't last very long, and the amount of blood lost is not great. Persistent, severe nosebleeds, however, require the attention of a nose and throat specialist, since occasionally the dilated nasal veins rupture and will need to be cauterized.

• This nasal congestion usually begins early on in pregnancy and tends to ease up somewhat in the later months. It may be confused with other types of nasal congestion such as allergies, overmedication, and chronic sinusitis.

•Before taking anything by mouth or by nose, it would be wise to check first—both as to the cause of congestion and the safety of medications.

Congestion of veins in the ear canals produces a feeling that resembles the effect of rapid descent in an airplane, or the stopped-up feeling you get in your ears after swimming. The unfortunate difference is that in pregnancy the sensation is persistent. Various drugs and drops have been used, but with transient and poor results. Most often the condition, once it develops, persists off and on until delivery and then is gone. What isn't?

Prenatal Fetal Testing

The ability to discern fetal abnormalities (or their absence) in early pregnancy has awakened a great deal of interest among clinicians as well as researchers. Thus, ultrasound evaluations, combined with certain chemical tests, have come to the forefront in this area. Most of the testing takes place late in the first trimester or early in the second—although as knowledge grows and tests improve, testing has been pushed back to even earlier days. This is a very fluid field, and changes will continue at a rapid pace.
Here are some of the basics:

•**Ultrasound.** Ultrasound is a fundamental tool in this arena. As it becomes more and more refined, accurate, and clear, it is being used to show defects in the spinal cord and brain so that early on we can see spina bifida, meningoceles, anencephaly (absence of the brain), and other treacherous nervous system disorders. Ultrasound also often reveals abnormalities of the heart, the digestive system, the extremities, the face, and other organ systems. It also reveals fetal growth restriction in the very early weeks of pregnancy— restrictions that generally indicate a high risk of chromosomal abnormalities. Ultrasound procedures are risk-free.

•**Amniocentesis.** This procedure is mentioned throughout the book and is indeed used at all stages of pregnancy and for a variety of procedures and tests. Early amniocentesis takes place in the first trimester or the early second trimester. Under ultrasound guidance, a needle is inserted through the anesthetized maternal abdominal wall into the uterus and on into the amniotic sac that envelops the fetus. Amniotic fluid is then withdrawn (the fetus quickly replaces it) and sent off for chromosomal analysis—a procedure that may take as long as 40 days. The risk of abortion is not great, but the laboratories have up to a 10 percent failure rate.

• **Chorionic villus sampling (CVS).** CVS involves entering the uterus through the cervical canal and siphoning away a piece of the placental tissue (the chorion) in order to submit it for chromosomal analysis. Like amniocentesis, it carries an abortion risk, as well as a similar laboratory failure rate, but results may be obtained much more rapidly (24–48 hours) and much larger tissue samples are obtained. Another important plus for CVS is that the risk in a subsequent therapeutic abortion is reduced because it can be done earlier in pregnancy than amniocentesis.

• **Embryoscopy.** This procedure is highly experimental at the moment, and I mention it only because you may hear about it. This is an approach that directly visualizes the embryo or fetus within the uterus. God knows what it will yield!

• **Alpha-fetoprotein (AFP).** This protein substance should not appear in the fetal circulation after the spinal cord has closed. When it gets into the fetal circulation because of certain spinal-closure abnormalities, it enters the maternal circulation as well, and we find, therefore, a maternal serum alpha-fetoprotein blood level (MSAFP). The MSAFP test has become a part of routine prenatal care and helps us to anticipate and manage certain developmental abnormalities—one of which is Down's syndrome.

• **MSAFP plus HCG** (remember?—human chorionic gonadotropin) **plus unconjugated estriol (E3) test.** Usually taken between the 18th and 25th week, this triad of maternal biochemical blood levels is a multiple screening test for Down's syndrome. It is 60 percent accurate in women under 35, and up to 89 percent accurate in women over 35. Other biochemical markers—including CA 125, the well-known ovarian cancer test—are all being studied to try to get the predictive value of this screen to a higher level.

These, then, are the major tests available to us at present for early fetal study. More are on the way. None are any simpler!

Prenatal Sex Determination

With the prenatal fetal testing methods available, it is clear that the sex of a fetus can be easily and certainly established. This information belongs to the mother, and she must be told—unless she wishes not to be. That sometimes is the case.

If the mother wishes to terminate the pregnancy for sex selection purposes alone, her physician is ethically bound not to participate in its destruction. If she chooses to go to an abortion center, that must be totally her decision.

Under certain genetic circumstances, however, a pregnancy termination may be considered as an appropriate resolution. As an example, male infants of a mother who carries the hemophilia gene will have a 50–50 chance of developing the disease. Other sex-linked genetic disorders can lead to similar management decisions.

More Pregnant Pauses

- The incidence of twins is decreasing worldwide. No one knows why.

- In 70 percent of American twins, two eggs are involved. In Japan it is the exact reverse. No one knows why.

- A head-on collision between two cars each going only 10 miles per hour will increase the weight of a newborn baby by 20 G forces. This would give the child an apparent and actual weight of 150 pounds! Few mothers can restrain that load. So after delivery, buckle up your baby, too. Be sure he or she is buckled up in a proper restraint.

- In a recent triplet pregnancy, the first infant delivered at the 23rd week. The pregnancy was maintained, and the two other infants delivered at 37½ weeks— 99 days later!

- Insomnia frequently plagues pregnant women who travel east through several time zones. You should snooze on arrival and thereafter try to avoid naps until your system adjusts. Avoid melatonin—a drug often used to manage jet lag.

- Twin-twin transfusion syndromes occur when one twin steals blood from its wombmate. This happens through conjoining blood vessels in the placenta, and it can be deadly. A new technique may provide the answer to this problem. It involves entering the uterus with a fetoscope, locating the placental vessels involved in the theft, and then lasering them shut.

- About 6 percent of all women seen in an emergency room are pregnant and don't know it.

- The power of a placebo is amazing. When verbally reinforced by the giver, a placebo shot, pill, or treatment can positively affect 30 percent of the takers. Thus, placebo power must be taken into account in any treatment or medication research trial. During a study in another country, the exact same placebo tablet, given to a group of separated volunteers, effectively increased or decreased their depressive symptoms depending entirely upon what they were told it would do!

Diary

My Fifth Month

Problems_____

_____

Medications_____

_____

_____

Rate of baby movement on a scale of 1–10_____

_____

_____

_____

Baby moved? When?_____

_____

_____

What's going on in the world?_____

_____

_____

_____

What's going on in my life?_____

_____

_____

_____

My thoughts and feelings_____

_____

_____

_____

Doctor's appointment_____

_____

_____

Questions to ask_____

Six

My Sixth Lunar Month

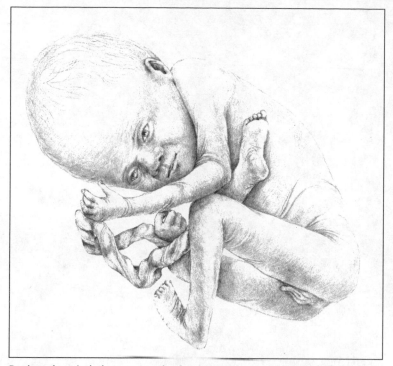

During the sixth lunar month, fetal growth picks up and at the end of this time it will weigh about 1.25 pounds (560 grams). Its head is still the largest body part. Protective fat under the skin increases but it remains wrinkled. Eyebrows and eyelashes are present, and the eyes open and close. Further, the mouth opens and amniotic fluid is regularly swallowed as a part of the amniotic circulation. If born at such a premature time, this infant can survive in a neonatal intensive care unit.

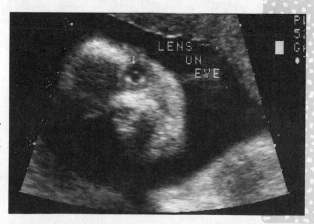

On ultrasound, a fair amount of the total body can still be seen, and in the remarkable cone-down view, one open eye is visible.

You are now entering the sixth lunar month of your pregnancy: the 20th to the 24th weeks. As you can see in the illustration that opens this chapter, your baby weighs only about a pound and a quarter. And yet, if by some catastrophe the baby should be born at this time, he or she would make every effort to live. The newly deposited fat under the skin would help to insulate the baby, who would also make gasping efforts. Survival is possible—even likely nowadays—in a neonatal intensive-care environment. A child weighing 14 ounces at birth has survived. Incredible, but true!

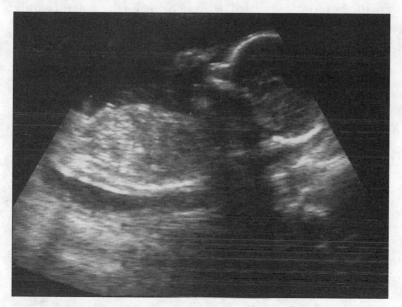

This is an ultrasound at 23 weeks.

At this stage, the baby moves inside you with a great deal more vigor. Since it is somewhat more difficult to get about because of the increasing size of your lower abdomen, you'd better be a little more careful about the way you move and the placement of steps and throw rugs, and now is the time to start wearing your heels—any heels—only on rare occasions.

Some companies used to suggest retirement about now. In a normal work environment, as we have already seen, this is no longer necessary or defensible. In employment that involves physical hazards, it may be necessary to terminate work at an earlier time or to accept transfer to a less physically demanding type of work. Under such circumstances, an employee's benefits and seniority will prevail in the future.

Also—the guy who brought you to this dance should now be attending some prenatal classes with you.

Intrauterine Growth Retardation (IUGR)

Although 8 percent of all babies delivered in the United States weigh less than 2,500 grams (5 lb., 8 oz.) and are, therefore, premature by definition, they are not all premature by actual dates. They are simply small for their gestational age and suffer from intrauterine growth retardation (IUGR). Further, of those infants born weighing more than 2,500 grams—and, therefore, not premature by definition—some 5 percent may also actually be growth-retarded because their weight is significantly below what their pregnancy duration demands. Thus, a child born at full term and weighing only 2,600 grams is a victim of IUGR for some important reason—known or unknown at the time.

There are two general categories of IUGR. The first is symmetrical: The whole body is reduced equally in size. The second is asymmetrical: The body is generally reduced to a greater degree than is the head. Symmetrical growth reduction is usually associated with an inherited fetal condition that is genetic in nature, but it may also be due to an injury sustained by the infant early in pregnancy, most likely from a systemic infection such as rubella or cytomegalovirus (see TORCH Syndrome in chapter 4).

Asymmetrical growth retardation in the fetus is a complication of certain maternal cardiovascular diseases, such as high blood pressure; maternal age (very old or very young); substance abuse, such as cigarettes, drugs, alcohol, or street drugs; chronic maternal lung disease; severe anemia; and certain less common maternal conditions.

The environment also apparently plays a role in IUGR; small babies are found at higher altitudes and in areas where expectant mothers are exposed to toxic substances (the Love Canal, for instance). Finally, multiple pregnancy will clearly produce IUGR, as will certain disorders of the placenta.

If a doctor suspects IUGR, close observation of fetal growth is very important. When maternal abdominal enlargement fails to keep up with the pregnancy dates, ultrasound study is indicated. Not only does ultrasound establish the diagnosis, it differentiates between the two types of IUGR and can further assess fetal health by providing a biophysical profile (see the appendix). Other diagnostic tools and procedures are used to detect and follow IUGR, but none is as reliable as ultrasound.

IUGR is managed by providing the infant with the best internal environment possible for the remainder of its time in the uterus. Such management includes extra maternal bed rest, adequate nutrition, cessation of substance abuse when possible, and removal of any damaging environmental factors. Close observation of fetal well-being and regular testing for fetal stress and distress are important. (Again, see the appendix). It is, unfortunately, often necessary to empty the uterus early if evidence of greatly reduced placental reserves or increasing fetal distress is shown. In such cases, labor must be watched very closely for further fetal distress. There is a higher incidence of delivery by cesarean section in some cases of IUGR.

The long-term outcome for these babies depends upon the initiating factor—that is, whatever is responsible for the IUGR in the first place—but generally, symmetrically growth-retarded infants remain small as infants and children and also exhibit continued neurological abnormalities. On the other hand, asymmetrically growth-retarded infants are more likely to catch up on their growth after birth and have fewer neurological complications.

In chapter 3, we discussed a form of IUGR that takes place in very early pregnancy and has been demonstrated only with the advent of advanced ultrasound. In these very early cases, embryo growth retardation is due to severe genetic disturbances, and survival—even to the fetal stage—is not possible.

Hypertension of Pregnancy

Hypertension of pregnancy, also known as pregnancy-induced hypertension (PIH), and known for centuries as preeclampsia or toxemia, has in the past contributed heavily to maternal and fetal mortality and disability. Although it is still a major problem and we still do not understand its basic cause, modern medical management has greatly reduced the risks to both mother and baby. Just to complicate this discussion as we move along, all three terms—PIH, preeclampsia, and toxemia—will be used interchangeably, since they refer to the same disorder.

What is it? PIH is a disorder limited almost exclusively to the last half of pregnancy, and mainly to the last ten weeks. It generally strikes young women having their first baby; older women in any pregnancy; women with preexisting high blood pressure, kidney disease, or diabetes; and, in particular, overweight women in a disadvantaged socioeconomic environment, who almost certainly also exhibit chronic malnutrition. (Note, though, that some socioeconomically *advantaged* women are also chronically malnourished—but by choice.) PIH is characterized by a triad of symptoms—namely, high blood pressure (hypertension), swelling of the tissues (edema), and albumin in the urine (proteinuria).

Why does it occur? A limitless number of theories have been advanced. This tells you something about our knowledge of PIH. Something that tells us even more is the bare icon adorning the ornate fretwork above the entrance to the famed Chicago Lying-in Hospital—an icon that is awaiting the name of the person who finally unearths the fundamental cause of PIH. It has been there for almost a century—and remains bare. Yet all people who work with the disorder agree that it is strictly limited to (human) pregnancy, that it is almost always restricted to the last half of pregnancy, and that it is apparently precipitated by an inadequate maternal blood supply to the placenta. One of its major dangers, then, is a reduction in blood flow (ischemia) to the placenta and the fetus, both of which feel this onslaught; in a reflex maneuver, the placenta puts out a substance to raise maternal blood pressure and, therefore, increase the pumping pressure of blood to itself and to the fetus. Sadly, it doesn't work very long, and the abnormal condition is only worsened, as is the fetal blood supply. So the vicious cycle continues, putting the fetus in distress and jeopardy. Moreover, ischemic damage to maternal organ systems can be overwhelming and permanent—it can even take the mother's life. When pregnancy is over, the placenta gone, and the disease abates and disappears, the surviving mother may be left with permanent high blood pressure, kidney disease, or other crippling problems.

This dangerous disorder begins, then, sometime in the second half of pregnancy—at least, that is when the signs and symptoms first arise. Usually it is mild at this time, with slight elevations of the blood pressure and equally slight general swelling and proteinuria. Under treatment, it may stay that way, or it may advance over time to severe preeclampsia. Very rarely, no matter how well managed, it will advance to full-blown eclampsia—a stage, characterized by convulsions, that requires immediate delivery.

Here is a recap of PIH:

- It is a condition, of unknown cause, that usually occurs after the 20th week of pregnancy.

- It is characterized by hypertension (high blood pressure), proteinuria (protein in the urine), and generalized swelling (edema).

- Despite adequate treatment, it may progress from mild to moderate to severe, and even to eclampsia (convulsions).

- The disorder generally strikes young women with their first pregnancy, older mothers with any pregnancy, mothers with preexisting hypertension, diabetes, kidney disease, or obesity, and those who are malnourished and economically disadvantaged.

•The disorder can induce profound fetal and maternal damage—
particularly if it is allowed to continue unchecked and untreated.

The Treatment of PIH

The ultimate treatment of this disorder is to get rid of the placenta. Thus, the cure lies in the delivery. This is no major management problem should PIH strike within a few weeks of full term. After adequate stabilization, the induction of labor or a cesarean section—whichever approach is obstetrically recommended—will get rid of the placenta.

Unfortunately, PIH usually mounts its attack well before full term. Here is the approach under those circumstances:

•The mother is very closely observed. Sometimes this requires a period of hospital observation to establish the blood pressure range and the daily degree of proteinuria and weight change, as well as to monitor the disorder's response to bed rest and/or medication. In more severe cases, prolonged hospital observation and treatment may be necessary.

•A very compliant mother may be managed at home—provided that she follows strict guidelines and promptly reports any symptom changes. Compliance involves frequent blood pressure checks, daily urine testing, weighing, and bed rest except for bathroom and eating excursions. Bed rest, lying on one side or the other, is a very important therapeutic weapon. Uterine blood flow is increased by this boring and difficult sojourn. Medication and dietary programs must be followed exactly.

•Careful fetal monitoring for activity and growth is obligatory during this difficult time. The intrauterine environment produced by PIH is often hostile to healthy fetal growth and development. This care involves stress and nonstress testing, biophysical profiling, and perhaps amniocentesis (see the appendix). An infant who appears reactive and normally growing is very reassuring. IUGR, however, is a common complication.

•Once the pregnancy approaches 37 weeks in a mild case, induction of labor may be undertaken as soon as the cervix is favorable for that procedure. If the case remains mild, we can wait a bit for the cervix to become more favorable—soft, thin, and somewhat open.

•When the preeclampsia is severe, we try to get the pregnancy to at least 34 weeks before attempting delivery. This is not always possible, even with the most meticulous management, and so delivery must be undertaken. The maturation of the infant's lungs may be hastened by predelivery cortisone—if there is time.

•If convulsions should strike, we are then dealing with eclampsia and immediate delivery is indicated, no matter what the stage of pregnancy or how well the infant is prepared. "Immediate delivery" must allow time for convulsion control and stabilization of the mother's condition insofar as possible while delivery preparations are being completed. Fortunately, eclampsia is a rare apocalypse.

It is worth pointing out again how important bed rest becomes in the management of PIH and its complications. Medications are often provided for the control of blood pressure and fluid retention, depending upon the extent of the disorder.

These treatment outlines are just that—outlines. Your own obstetrician will tailor your treatment to your needs and to the appropriate planning for your particular case should this devilish condition plague your pregnancy. PIH induces other pregnancy complications—all of which your obstetrician is aware of and ready to manage. One of the most worrisome is the HELLP syndrome, which we will look at next.

It is important to know that women who have had preeclampsia in their first pregnancy are more likely (15–20 percent) to have it again in a subsequent pregnancy. Moreover, preeclampsia increases the risk of future chronic hypertension and renal disease. You must weigh the potential for these problems in consultation with your obstetrician in order to arrive at your future reproductive goals. It may be important to have certain cardiovascular and renal studies undertaken in order to arrive at a rational decision.

Various experimental programs are under way to test certain theories concerning the prevention of PIH. Two agents being widely tested include calcium and the once lowly, now mighty aspirin. Their testing, as I said, is based upon certain theories of PIH causation. The value of either one is yet to be established, although some studies seem to indicate a protective role for aspirin.

Is there anything that you can do to prevent PIH from endangering your pregnancy—and you? The most important step in protecting both yourself and your baby should be taken before you become pregnant. Adequate nutritional habits and weight control are critical. If you enter pregnancy well nourished and within your normal BMI, you have much going for you. Should you be burdened with chronic hypertension, renal disease, diabetes, or some other contributing systemic disorder, you and your physician need to establish tight control over these problems before you do the deed. Nutrition, weight control, and adequate rest while you are pregnant will go a long way toward protecting you and your child.

HELLP!

Depending upon which research study we read, HELLP may complicate anywhere from 2 to 12 percent of the very severe cases of preeclampsia. It most often occurs before delivery, but up to 30 percent will appear anywhere from the first few hours up to a week after delivery. HELLP is considered a very major complication of severe preeclampsia. We do not know what generates it in certain cases of PIH, but fortunately, it is not often encountered.

What does HELLP mean? Well, it is an acronym for the major disorders that it spawns, namely:

- **H**emolysis (blood destruction)
- **EL**evated and abnormal liver function tests
- **L**ow **P**latelet counts

With these abnormalities, the syndrome, unfortunately, mimics many other illnesses. Blood pressures are not necessarily much elevated, adding to the diagnostic difficulty. The symptoms are also often vague and non-specific—nausea, upper abdominal pain, weakness, and edema are usually present early on. Later, jaundice and spontaneous bleeding from the gums, kidneys, and intestines may appear, along with abnormal liver and blood findings. Once the diagnosis is confirmed, prompt delivery is almost always necessary. If it happens to attack after delivery, it is generally short-lived and responds to proper therapeutic measures. Since HELLP, like PIH, tends to recur in future pregnancies, its risk must also be considered in counseling a mother who is contemplating another pregnancy.

Amniotic Fluid Problems

Amniotic fluid begins to appear at about the eighth week of gestation, which is the same time when the fetus begins to urinate. That is what amniotic fluid mainly consists of—fetal urine. The volume of amniotic fluid increases until the 34th week and thereafter gradually declines, so that at full term there may be 800–1,500 cc's (2¾ oz–1½ qt) available for the infant to float and thrash around in.

Now, where does all the fetal urine go? Well, it is turned over very rapidly into the maternal circulation—a complete changeover takes place about every 20 minutes under normal circumstances. Fetal swallowing also contributes significantly to the circulation of amniotic fluid.

There are a number of conditions in pregnancy that can lead to excessive amniotic fluid (hydramnios) or too little (oligohydramnios)—both of which conditions may signal other problems.

Conditions associated with hydramnios are:

- diabetes
- Rh and other blood sensitizations
- twins or more
- fetal abnormalities
- certain TORCH infections
- other unknown causes

Complications of hydramnios may be:

- premature labor
- placental separation
- premature rupture of membranes
- prolapse of the umbilical cord
- abnormal fetal position
- abnormal labor
- postpartum bleeding

Conditions associated with oligohydramnios are:

- fetal anomalies
- high blood pressure
- drugs of all kinds
- overdue pregnancy
- certain autoimmune disorders

Complications of oligohydramnios may be:

- fetal and cord compression
- intrauterine fetal death
- fetal distress in labor
- maternal problems

The volume of amniotic fluid can be determined with accuracy by repeated ultrasound screenings. The clinical management of amniotic problems depends on ultrasound findings, other clinical findings, the judgment of the physician, and the concordance of the mother.

More on Amniotic Fluid

Under many circumstances, and at various times throughout pregnancy, amniotic fluid may be withdrawn for laboratory testing. Fetal maturity, Rh sensitization, genetic status, early fetal structural disorders, intrauterine infections—these conditions and more can be clarified from study of this fluid. Removing amniotic fluid is a comparatively safe procedure when done with ultrasound guidance. Local anesthesia in the maternal abdominal wall prevents most discomfort.

Amniotic fluid may also be drawn off as necessary in certain cases of hydramnios. It also may be added to by a process called *amnioinfusion*. This procedure may be used during a labor in which the amount of amniotic fluid is reduced for some reason. This reduction may compress the umbilical cord during labor contractions, with resultant fetal distress. Amnioinfusion is still not widely used, since its benefits are not absolutely established. When it is done during labor, the procedure involves running warm glucose solution through a catheter inserted into the uterine cavity through the cervix. As always with invasive procedures, there are risks and complications about which mothers need to be informed.

Meconium consists of the infant bowel contents that normally spill but very slightly and intermittently from the rectum and into amniotic fluid—not in enough volume to even discolor its clear appearance. Certain kinds of fetal distress, however, paralyze the anal sphincter, which then allows much more meconium into the amniotic fluid. Thus, if meconium-stained amniotic fluid appears during labor—once membranes are ruptured—we often have an indicator of fetal distress. This observation is not always correct, however, and must be used in conjunction with other observations and tests. One obvious false-positive meconium appearance is during breech (bottom first) labors. In this situation, the baby's lower abdomen is compressed by laboring through the pelvis and thus meconium squirts out.

Relaxin Symptoms

In every pregnancy, a variable amount of a hormone substance called relaxin is secreted, probably by the anterior pituitary gland. This hormone substance has but one purpose, and that is to relax the ligaments around your pelvis and hips so that they will stretch more easily during labor and thus ease your baby's trip. An unfortunate side effect of this ligament relaxation, however, is a feeling of pelvic instability. You may feel as if your hips are going to come out of their sockets, particularly when you first get out of a chair or out of bed. This relaxation of the joints is responsible for the "crick" and "catches" in your hips (not your back) and for the pain you often feel in the bottom of your abdomen as the pubic bones begin to separate. Relaxin also slackens your other joints, and this is why, in advising you on exercise, we suggested that your joints be spared excessive activity (see pages 47–53).

Little can be done to ward off this feeling, but like so many other things we have spoken about, it will disappear soon after you deliver. Promises, promises!

Varicose Veins

We have talked about the pressure on rectal veins caused by the growing baby. This pressure can cause hemorrhoids—anal or rectal varicose veins. Pressure is also transmitted to blood vessels in the lower extremities, producing a tendency toward varicose—or swollen—veins. These may become more of a problem with each pregnancy. Pressure increases as pregnancy progresses, and not only do the veins become swollen, but there is some risk of complications—such as clotting. For this reason, and for long-term health and cosmetic reasons, it is important to take care of such swollen veins if they develop during your pregnancy. First of all, never wear constricting circular garters to hold your hose up, and never roll your hose. (I don't think anyone does that anymore, but if you do, don't.) Second, try to avoid standing for long periods of time without rest or without moving around. Third, whenever the veins become a problem, wear some form of supportive hose. Relatively inexpensive, indeed almost attractive, hose for pregnancy that gives adequate support for most women can now be bought at maternity, drug, or department stores. If more help is needed, your doctor will order special supportive hose for you at a surgical supply house. They look like cigar wrappers, but they work! Further:

- If significant clots do form in leg veins, there will almost always be swelling and pain in that extremity—sure signs that you need your obstetrician's help.

- Remember, if you have to sit still for any length of time—as in a long turbulent flight—move and exercise your leg muscles at regular intervals. Get out of a car and walk around. Stand up from a desk and go get a decaf, anything. Even if you are forced to lie in bed because of preeclampsia or because you are expecting a multiple brood, exercise those legs!

•Remember that earlier we saw how all your veins will dilate somewhat everywhere on your skin. Thus, you will see them stand out more on your arms and even mottle the palms of your hands. This is a hormonal effect that goes when your baby goes. Sure!

Particular Problems of Younger and Older Expectant Mothers

If you have been paying attention, you already know about such conditions as high-risk pregnancy, PIH, IUGR, the whole bit, and you are now properly depressed about all the things that can happen to you as you wander down the maternity trail. Well, let's continue that litany by checking out the problems of younger and older mothers.

Here are the most common problems presented in adolescent and senior pregnancies:

The Minors

•incomplete body growth of the expectant mother herself, who is therefore competing with her baby for nutrients, to the detriment of both

•more low-birth-weight-for-date babies (IUGR)

•greatly increased incidence of premature labor and premature infants

•increased disproportion between the baby's head and the small maternal pelvis

•greater incidence of PIH

•more cesarean sections

•more nutritional problems and anemia

•tendency to not seek competent help or follow advice

The Majors

Recognizing that a mother of some 63 years has recently and successfully delivered a healthy girl, we need to be careful about whom we designate as an "older" mother and what chronological age we dare to suggest is the start-up point! Modern fertility experts are regularly increasing the coterie of mature-mother pregnancies by assisted-reproductive procedures. Not only that, they are regularly increasing the number of plural-pregnancy formations with such procedures. In another vein, women are delaying pregnancy until their later years in order to consummate career goals. So both the majors and the minors are playing more active roles in the reproductive field.

Regardless of all these changes taking place, obstetricians continue to cast 35 years as the starting point for a mature pregnancy. Here are some events that begin to multiply about that time:

- greater incidence of medical complications such as diabetes, hypertension, and renal disease

- greater incidence of congenital disorders in the newborn

- labor that is more likely to be ineffectual and require help

- higher cesarean section rate

- risks of the whole gamut of obstetrical complications in multiparous older mothers (women who have had many children)

- possible permanent and irreversible effects in older women of the complications of prolonged smoking and other body abuse

From the obstetrician's point of view, it may be easier to take care of the older mothers-to-be than the younger ones. They seem to realize better what is at stake, follow advice much more closely, and do everything they can to protect their pregnancy—and themselves.

In spite of reliable birth control, reliable emergency contraception, and abortion on demand, there is still a very high proportion of unwanted pregnancies in our country, the vast majority of which occur in teenage girls. It is estimated that 1 girl in 10 becomes a mother before she graduates from high school—about 1 million this year, of whom some 600,000 will go on to deliver. It is fortunately true that this rate is slowly declining, but at the same time the rate of unwed teenage mothers is regularly rising. Adolescent mothers are beset not only by the problems I have mentioned but also by a host of fundamental emotional problems associated with having to adapt to their new role as a mother before they have adapted to the role of a growing girl. As one of them put it, "One minute I was a running, ripping, hopping, jumping 14-year-old girl. Then I got pregnant."

Going from age 13 to 20 in nine months is a very long, hard jump. These youngsters are also often confronted by the problem of not having an understanding relationship with their parents, physician, or counselor. Such an unfortunate mother is many times advised to have an abortion when she doesn't want one, to have a baby when she doesn't want one, to marry when she doesn't want to, to not marry when she wants to, and to give up something or someone whom she loves dearly. It is sometimes difficult for adults to remember that the desires of love and the sorrows of loss are felt just as greatly by youngsters as by adults. They are not forgotten any sooner or with any less trauma. They just occur at an earlier age.

Pregnant adolescents need a great deal of help, that is certain. It would take a separate chapter to outline their needs and a whole book to answer them. Here, however, are some suggestions:

- Search out an adult in the health care field—your doctor, a nurse-practitioner, a trained social worker—someone to whom you can relate, in whom you can confide, and with whom you can bond. You will be surprised by how easy they are to find and how eager they are to help. Share your problems with them, and they will give you the best help you can get.

- Eat carefully. Avoid junk food and salt. A recent study shows that 30 percent of all high school students tested had abnormally high blood cholesterol levels and that one in eight was overweight. Don't jeopardize your growth and your baby's growth.

- If you smoke, quit. If you don't, don't start. Avoid alcohol and drugs of any kind for any purpose.

- Take your vitamins and minerals as given to you.

- Continue to strengthen your relationship with your bonding person, and listen to the advice you get. That is one of the most important things I can tell you.

Pets—Out Damned Spot!

Most American households harbor one or more pets. The emotional and physical benefits derived from the human-animal bond are well recognized, and the therapeutic value of the bond has been well established and documented. On the other hand, domestic animals that you have raised and loved can, and do, harbor conditions that may affect you during your pregnancy and, indeed, at any time.

The common household dog that provides a great deal of companionship and protection may also be host to a number of parasites that can infect the whole family. The most common of these offenders is the pinworm, which is not a serious infestation itself but is easily spread throughout a whole family. When this takes place, everyone—human and canine—must be purged of the parasite. Under ordinary circumstances, there is no problem in having the whole family take the necessary indicated medication. However, such medication should not be taken by a pregnant woman, particularly during the first trimester of her pregnancy. Thus, she will have to wait to rid herself of the scourge, meanwhile possibly reinfecting family members who have already been treated.

Dogs harbor a number of other organisms that can and are transmitted to humans. The most serious of these is rabies, which presents a particular dilemma during pregnancy (see the discussion of immunization on pages 135–138). It is important that you keep your dog's immunizations current for this and, of course, many other reasons.

Dogs are the home of many fleas and often many ticks. Besides being a bloody nuisance, ticks can carry serious human infections. Your veterinarian now has tablets or applications that, used on a monthly basis, will rid your dog of both parasites.

Cats are another, more serious problem. Scratches and bites from household cats are a common occurrence. Moreover, cats are innate predators and are likely to be exposed to anything infectious or toxic that has injured their prey. Rodents, which are a significant portion of their prey, can be infested with any number of deadly or crippling organisms. Moreover, since cats lick their paws, and therefore their claws, these areas are frequently a source of infection, as are their bites. One particular bacteria that is a normal resident of the cat's mouth can produce fever and lymph gland enlargements, which are similar to symptoms of plague or tularemia. Finally, and of great importance during pregnancy, cats are one major source of human infections with toxoplasmosis, which has a devastating effect on pregnancy (see TORCH syndrome in chapter 4). The other toxoplasmosis carrier is poorly cooked meat.

It may sound from all of this that I don't think much about cats; that is not true. I think about them a great deal, and I think they should be banished during pregnancy. That is easy to say, in practice often impossible, and, in the opinion of some observers, not nearly as important as the proper cooking of all meats. If you do keep a cat, at least an inside cat, avoid close contact if you can, including tender licks and playful scratches. Let someone else manage the litter boxes. Avoid outside cats like the plague!

Although dogs and cats are the usual representatives of the animal world in our households, numerous other species may be found, including fish, birds, reptiles, and rodents. Since we may have frequent intimate contact with most of these communal inhabitants of our domestic environment, we must not overlook their attendant hazards.

As a general rule, do not make pets of, or approach, any wild animals or birds. They may harbor rabies, various viruses, bacterial infections, fungus, and, as we have noted, in the western United States, the plague. When all things are considered, your mate is probably your safest pet— but only by a slight margin!

Fresh Pregnant Pauses

- •At term, a healthy fetus can swallow 450 cc's of amniotic fluid daily. This coincides with the amount of milk that a newborn infant can daily swallow the first few weeks after birth.

- •Maternal smoking during pregnancy increases the risk of stillbirth or infant death within a month after birth by 20 to 35 percent, and increases the risk of premature labor by 36 to 50 percent.

- •The famous Chicago Lying-in Hospital, built early in this century, had as its first master the equally famous obstetrician Joseph B. DeLee. He directed the architects to place a series of finials with shields or icons along the upper fretwork of the hospital, each to be inscribed with the name of a famous leader in the advancement of care for women. He was the doctor who ordered that one space be left blank for the person who eventually discovers the cause of hypertension of pregnancy. As I told you, it is still blank.

- •Some strange facts about preeclampsia:
  Women who cohabit with the father of their child for over a year preceding conception have a greatly reduced risk of preeclampsia.
  Women who switch partners between pregnancies are at a greater risk for PIH.
  Women who conceive using donor sperm insemination are also at greater risk.

- •Laparoscopic surgery is apparently safe during pregnancy—even in the last trimester. Most commonly the procedure is done for gall bladder removal, but appendectomies and certain other operations are thus accomplished. Studies indicate that laparoscopic surgery, when possible, is safer than open abdominal operations.

- •Doctors—like everyone else—have some unusual names. For instance, in our country there are at least 18 doctors named Doctor. Thus, we have some "Dr. Doctor" doctors. There are some named Fix, Cure, and Heal—as well as Klutz, Croak, Blunt, and Blewitt. Also in practice we have an anesthetist named Gass, an orthopedist named Knee, a psychiatrist named Couch, and a dermatologist named Rash! There are also a few Dr. Nurses (from *Journal of the American Medical Association,* December 1992).

Diary

My Sixth Month

Problems_____

_____

Medications_____

_____

_____

Rate of baby movement on a scale of 1–10_____

_____

_____

Natural childbirth classes_____

_____

_____

_____

What's going on in the world?_____

_____

_____

_____

What's going on in my life?_____

_____

_____

_____

My thoughts and feelings_____

_____

_____

_____

Doctor's appointment_____

_____

_____

Questions to ask_____

Seven

My Seventh Lunar Month

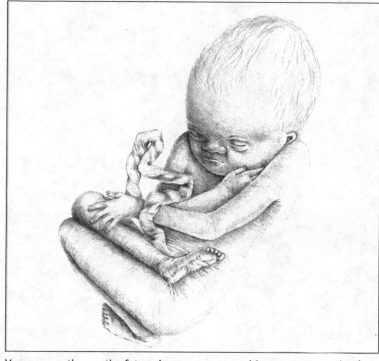

Your seventh-month fetus is now approaching two pounds (900 grams) and is busy waving his hands, sucking his thumb, or kicking you everywhere! The covering skin is now smoothing out and is coated with a waxy substance called "vernix caseosa" to protect it against its fluid environment. Its eyelids continue to open and close— although there is nothing to see. The fetus can hear and your young one recognizes your voice. Be careful!

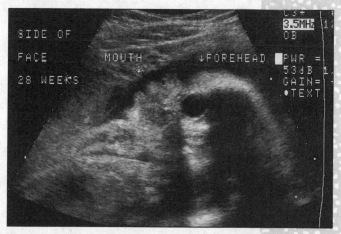

The ultrasound clearly shows some thumb-sucking. A close-up reveals an open mouth and what appears to be an empty eye socket. Not to worry—it is just a closed lid.

These are the 24th to the 28th weeks of your pregnancy. There are still 24 hours to a day, but you may feel like you are up to 28. If, by chance, you should begin labor and your baby is born at this time, it has a good chance of surviving in an intensive-care nursery and of being healthy. Winston Churchill was born during the seventh month—and born at home!

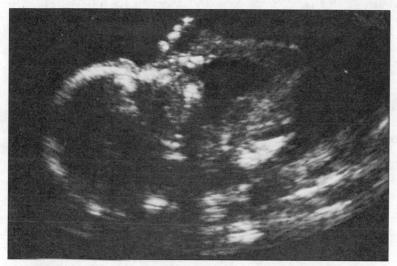

A 28-week fetus, lying placidly on its back and sucking it's thumb.

One of the entrenched pregnancy tales is that a child born at the end of the seventh month has a better chance of survival than one born at the end of the eighth month. This is absolutely incorrect and should be put to rest along with that other old tale "for every child a tooth"! One of the most important things to remember is that in a *normal* pregnancy, every day a child remains in the uterus until full term increases its chance of survival.

As for your symptoms, while everyone else is freezing, you'll be fanning yourself. Lying flat in bed may make you short of breath, and you may notice your heart fluttering (palpitations) from time to time, whether you are resting or working. All these things are normal. Where have you heard that before?

Heartburn and Other Digestive Disturbances

Perhaps you thought when you finished early pregnancy that eating was forevermore going to be an endless and joyous indulgence, within the limits dictated by your scales, your pocketbook, and your provider's temper. Your stomach may now be telling you otherwise. Heartburn may become a regular companion—it does in about 50 percent of all pregnancies. If you have never experienced heartburn before, it is a hot, irritating sensation in the lower chest, usually present after meals or before bedtime. It is worse if you have eaten fried or highly seasoned foods, which are not supposed to be on your table anyway, and you know it.

Heartburn at this time is related to changes in the physiology and anatomy of the lower esophagus, and it cannot be cured during pregnancy. It can, however, be temporarily relieved by the following:

- Avoid fried, greasy, or highly seasoned foods.

- Take frequent sips of (skim) milk or, better still, chew cracked ice.

- Take modern over-the-counter antacid preparations that do not contain sodium derivatives.

- Severe heartburn may be managed with drugs such as Tagamet and Axid. These drugs are very effective and may also be purchased over-the-counter. However, neither their safety nor their risk in pregnancy has been confirmed. You need to consult your obstetrician before resorting to these agents.

In late pregnancy, your stomach is pushed way up under your chest, thus often becoming congested and a very ineffective repository for food. Indigestion, nausea, and vomiting may result, particularly if you eat too much and too well. Therefore, it is important, as it was in early pregnancy, to avoid big meals and not to lie down after you eat—or, putting it another way, do not eat before you lie down.

A rare condition, diaphragmatic (epigastric, hiatus) hernia, produces severe, sometimes uncontrollable nausea and vomiting in late pregnancy and requires very special care. As with so much else, the hernia, the abdominal pressure, and the heartburn—all disappear with delivery. Everything disappears with delivery except the baby, the bills, and some of the bulges.

Pressure Symptoms

By this time, your friends have already given you blow-by-blow and push-by-push details about pressure symptoms in late pregnancy. Now you know what they were talking about and—for once—they were right. Just as the weight of the expanding uterus changes the position of the stomach and affects its ability to digest food, so the baby pushes against other abdominal organs and packs them up against your diaphragm. This pressure prevents the diaphragm from expanding adequately when you breathe, and thus you feel the shortness of breath that is so common in late pregnancy.

Sometime during the last month, your baby may drop rather suddenly into your pelvis. This so-called lightening does not always occur before the onset of labor, but if it does, you will experience great relief in your upper abdomen and chest. You will be able to breathe more easily and eat more readily without digestive disturbances, and by and large you will feel a great deal more comfortable. On the other hand, your baby may descend more slowly into the pelvis over a period of weeks, and the upper abdominal relief may thus be less striking. At any rate, what is no longer up is down, and the pressure in your lower abdomen and pelvis increases, causing you seemingly ceaseless trips to and from the bathroom. Have faith and endure. Relief is on the way!

Cesarean Section

The process of delivering a child by incision through the abdominal wall and the uterus has been known since prehistoric times, as indicated in early cave paintings in Africa. As recently as 200 years ago, a famous British obstetrician named William Smellie had this to say about cesarean section in his textbook on obstetrics:

> When a woman cannot be delivered by any of the methods hitherto prescribed and recommended in laborious and preternatural labors on account of narrowness or distortion of the pelvis into which it is sometimes impossible to introduce the hand—in such emergencies, if the woman is strong and of good habit of body, the cesarean operation is certainly advisable and ought to be performed because the mother and the child have no other chance to be saved. It is better to have recourse to an operation which *sometimes* succeeds than leave them both to inevitable death.

This was the state of cesarean operations at that time. It was mainly—almost exclusively—performed on women who were at the point of death or actually dead, with no hope of saving the mother, only of obtaining a live child. It had been thus since antiquity. When it was attempted on a living woman, she almost invariably died thereafter.

One hundred years later, the results were not much better. A textbook written at that time reported that three-quarters of the living women on whom the operation was performed subsequently died.

Today, of course, cesarean sections are a relatively safe operation; many hospitals in our country and elsewhere have *never* experienced a maternal death from the cesarean procedure. This improved safety record is due to modern surgical techniques, anesthesia, antibiotics, and blood replacement, as well as, in broad terms, a healthier population and an increasing store of obstetrical wisdom and judgment.

The operation, as we have seen, was known to very early African cultures as well as to the Greeks, the Egyptians, and the Chinese at the height of their cultures, but again, the operation was probably resorted to only when the mother was at the point of death or after her death. Pliny the Elder, the Roman naturalist, claimed in his writings that the renowned general Scipio, who defeated Hannibal, was the first person thus brought into the world. This is not so, but the operation's name is in fact derived from Roman culture. Because they had been cut out of their mother's womb, such Roman individuals were first termed *caesons* and afterward *caesares.* To quote directly from the Latin source, "Quia caeso matris utero in lucem prodiscunt," which roughly translates as: a child should be removed from the uterus if its mother should die in late pregnancy. This law was known initially as the *lex regia* and continued under the rule of the Caesars, thus acquiring the name *lex caesaria;* and those delivered in this manner became known as *caesares.* Julius Caesar is said to have been brought into the world this way, but it is erroneous to state that the name Caesar was given to him on this account or that the operation was named for him. And that's enough ancient history.

Modern reasons for cesarean sections include:

- previous cesarean section (see discussion of VBAC later in this chapter)

- certain maternal or fetal forms of distress during labor

- disproportion between the fetal head and the maternal pelvis

- abnormal infant presentation—a breech, for instance

- hemorrhage from a separated placenta

- certain medical disorders such as diabetes

- multiple pregnancy

These are the major reasons the cesarean operation is performed in modern obstetrics, but there are others. It is very important for us to understand that *none* of these indications is *absolute* and that a great deal of judgment is required in the section decision. A host of factors must be considered.

Types of Cesarean Section

Classical. This is the operation described through antiquity—a bold up-and-down incision in the lower abdominal wall, another bold up-and-down incision through the uterus, and, quickly, the operator is in and the child is out. Today the operation is rarely used, mainly being reserved for situations where extra rapid delivery is necessary. Examples might be when the mother dies suddenly—as in an accident—or when there is sudden severe fetal distress. Rarely, a classical incision may be necessary because a placenta previa (see page 51) covers the lower uterine surfaces where the modern incision is made. Why is the classical uterine incision seldom used? Mainly because it heals poorly and the risk of spontaneous rupture of the uterus in a future pregnancy is very real—even without labor. Moreover, future deliveries have to done using the same classical uterine incision, further weakening the uterus. To substitute a low cervical section in a future delivery would be adding one more scar to the already scarred uterus.

Low Cervical. This is the standard modern operation. The uterus is opened transversely in its very lowest segment. Under certain conditions—to be discussed shortly—future pregnancies may possibly be delivered vaginally.

Cesarean Hysterectomy. This operation combines a cesarean section with a following hysterectomy. The hysterectomy may be a planned procedure to remove, at one procedure, a diseased uterus as well as a child. An example might be an early noninvasive cervical cancer, but there are others. The uterus may also be removed at this time as an emergency tactic—such as when bleeding is uncontrollable or when the uterus has been irreparably ruptured.

There are several other rare types of cesarean sections that you may somehow hear about. A **Porro** section operation (which I have never seen and probably is never done anymore) was accomplished by removing the uterus with the baby still inside, then cutting the uterus open to remove the baby! It may have been an attempt to keep an infected uterine cavity—and baby—from infecting the mother and causing her to develop peritonitis. An **extra-peritoneal** section has been developed to do the same thing—to prevent the spread of infection from an involved uterus into the maternal peritoneal cavity. It is a tedious and difficult anatomical procedure and is almost always avoided nowadays by using an adequate antibiotic umbrella prior to surgery and continuing it thereafter.

Anesthesia for Cesarean Sections

There is a complete discussion of anesthesia in childbirth and of all the available techniques, as well as their benefits and risks, on pages 242–248.

Should you have a section, the type of pain relief used will most likely be decided by you, your doctor, and the anesthesiologist or anesthetist, who will all be working together for the greatest safety for you and your baby.

Cesarean Section Rate

At the end of World War II—which was not so long ago—the section rate in the United States was about 7 percent, and the maternal mortality resulting from, or associated with, sections was around 10 percent. Today our section rate is about 24 percent, and the associated maternal mortality rate has declined as rapidly as the section incidence has increased. There are multiple reasons for this remarkable increase in sections, among them:

- Sections have replaced difficult forceps vaginal deliveries.
- Sections have also replaced most breech (bottom first) deliveries.
- With the increased incidence of plural pregnancies, sections are more common.
- Teenage mothers, of whom we have an abundance, are more likely to have a small pelvis.
- Vaginal herpes lesions at term require a section delivery.
- Epidemic obesity is producing an epidemic of larger babies.
- The number of previous sections is increasing.
- Obstetricians have significant fears of malpractice suits.

There are many concerns about this escalating section rate, and many practitioners are trying to reduce the rate to some magical figure or percentage point. While that goal does not appear to be in sight at the moment, one reduction effort now being widely employed is called VBAC.

Vaginal Birth After a Cesarean Section (VBAC)

The greater number of VBACs being performed represents one potential solution to the ever-increasing number of cesarean sections in this country. Fully one-third of all sections are repeats, and it used to be an iron-clad rule that "once a section, always a section." This is true today only when the previous operation was a classical section—which, as you know, is seldom performed anymore—and when there are conditions that persist in each pregnancy—for example, a very contracted maternal pelvis. Studies now reveal that, following proper guidelines, some 50 to 80 percent of women who previously had a section may be delivered vaginally with less risk than a repeat section poses. Those guidelines are as follows:

1. No specific indication for a cesarean section should exist in the present pregnancy.

2. One or more previous sections should not rule out an attempted vaginal delivery.

3. If questions remain about the previous section, the case must be individually assessed and answers sought. Those questions include: What was the cause of the previous section? What type was done? Were there any maternal uterine infections afterward?

4. The hospital must have the resources to be able to respond instantly to an emergency and do a section within 30 minutes.

5. A physician who is capable of evaluating labor and performing a cesarean section must be readily available.

In November 1988, the American College of Obstetricians and Gynecologists held a major news conference to announce that VBAC was to be seen as a routine procedure. Since that time, many thousands of cases have been collected attesting to the relative safety of VBACs. Mind you, there are problems associated with the procedure—some of them very serious—and a certain number of VBAC attempts fail. Nevertheless, when the physician is skilled, the overall risks are not as great as those of a repeat section.

Further Cesarean Section Information

If VBAC is not an option, a healthy woman may undergo about as many repeat cesarean operations as the family budget will allow—providing there are no significant complications along the way. As many as *nine* have been recorded for one intrepid mother. It is important that each succeeding pregnancy be evaluated very, very closely.

It is also important to assess fetal maturity before doing an elective repeat section. This involves both clinical and laboratory determinations. Clinical signs include the date when the fetal heart was first heard, as well as evidence of uterine growth from at least the 16th week. Laboratory findings include records of early blood pregnancy testing and certain ultrasound determinations.

It usually takes about 45 minutes to perform an uncomplicated cesarean section. Certain complications can vastly extend this time.

Recovery from a section is usually quite rapid. Generally the patient experiences abdominal discomfort because, after all, abdominal surgery was performed. She also has gas pains for a day or so.

As a rule, the hospital stay is only a day or two longer than for a vaginal delivery, but more help time is necessary at home. The managed care industry has tried to throw section mothers out of the hospital the day after their operations, but legislation (and probably their wives and mothers) forced them to recant and drop their Klingon approach to us humanoids.

Heart Changes and Palpitations

Your heart is called upon to do a great deal of extra work during pregnancy. The volume of blood that it has to pump increases by 20 to 25 percent, and it becomes a great deal more difficult to circulate this blood because of the hemodynamics involved. For example, the growing baby exerts marked reverse pressure against the drainage of blood from your lower extremities. This is why expectant mothers who have heart disease must be watched very closely as pregnancy progresses.

The normal heart can take the added stress without any serious limitations whatsoever. It is moved out of position by the rising diaphragm and winds up considerably left of center. This sometimes makes your heartbeat more readily felt, and since your heart will occasionally beat much more rapidly (palpitations), the new experience may be somewhat frightening. In a normal heart, these changes are never dangerous and soon stop if ignored. In the presence of heart disease, however, very special instructions are given during pregnancy, and these must be followed closely.

One note of great interest: Women who have undergone heart surgery such as coronary bypass procedures, heart valve replacements, congenital defect corrections, and, yes, even heart transplants—all types have successfully delivered!

Leg Cramps

It is 4:00 A.M., and you have been to the bathroom ten times tonight, and even *The Late Late Show* is over, and you are sick of looking at ads for "buns-of-steel" exercise equipment or fail-proof food dehydrators—but that's all there is to watch. So you are trying to catch a few moments of delicious sleep when—zap!—it hits you. Your legs pull up in one tremendous cramp that throws you out of bed or causes you to writhe and kick and grab at your legs until your husband is convinced that you are possessed. What's happening now?

What's happening now is a tetanic contraction of your leg muscles due most likely to a disturbance of calcium metabolism, brought about by who knows what? But even though the disturbance is not completely understood, correction is at hand.

- •First of all, eliminate milk from your diet. As we have already noted, milk in large amounts is not now considered important during pregnancy—if your diet is otherwise adequate in protein and calcium and if you have been taking your vitamin/mineral supplements regularly. Milk is not necessarily a good source of calcium for pregnant women; in fact, it may prevent some calcium from getting into your system.

- •If eliminating milk fails to stop your leg cramps promptly, add extra calcium to your nutritional program. Tums and Rolaids are inexpensive sources of calcium replacement (read the labels). Some other sources, such as certain juices, contain added calcium citrate, which your system absorbs very completely. Look back to our dietary section for your calcium requirements and other supplemental sources.

- •When the cramps do occur, get up and move around. Massage your leg or let your husband do it, or get into a tub of hot water. But not with him.

Certain other muscular discomforts occur in late pregnancy, but these are generally due to the relaxation of ligaments and other supports of the pelvic bone, and they don't stab at you like the nighttime demons.

Rh Blood Disorders

In the past, a great deal was written about the Rh disorders that complicated pregnancy, often ending in fetal damage or destruction. With the advent of modern vaccination programs, serious Rh disorders have, blessedly, become exceedingly rare.

Here's what it's all about. The Rh factor is a protein substance in the blood of about 85 percent of all humans. They are therefore Rh-positive. The remaining 15 percent, lacking the Rh factor, are Rh-negative. The Rh factor, like the color of the eyes, is inherited. It does nothing and goes nowhere. It is important only during blood transfusions and during pregnancy. When a blood transfusion is to be given, it is important to match the Rh factors. Actually, an Rh-positive person can receive Rh-negative blood without any difficulty or reaction, but the reverse is certainly not true.

In pregnancy, trouble may arise when the father is Rh-positive and the mother Rh-negative. The unborn child, then, has an 85 percent chance of being Rh-positive. During pregnancy and more actively during delivery, some Rh-positive blood from the baby escapes into the circulation of its Rh-negative mother. Since this blood contains a foreign protein substance, the mother begins to build up antibodies against it. (This process is governed by the laws of immunity: A body tends to build antibodies against any foreign protein that appears within it—the basis for vaccinations and inoculations against diseases.) These antibodies are protective to their host—the mother. All would be fine, except that some of these antibodies can get back into the baby's circulation across the placenta and proceed to destroy the baby's blood cells, since they are antibodies against Rh-positive cells.

Since it usually takes a pregnancy and delivery to initiate the process, there is almost never any difficulty with the Rh factor in the first pregnancy because that pregnancy is the sensitizing one. But in subsequent pregnancies, if preventive vaccine has not been given, the baby may be born anemic, jaundiced, or, worst of all, dead. However, there are now tests that can be performed on an Rh-negative mother's blood (Coombs' test), as well as other procedures involving amniotic fluid that can determine whether this sensitization is taking place.

One common amniotic fluid test is a spectrophotometric analysis, which measures the optical density of amniotic fluid. The density becomes abnormal when blood pigment (bilirubin) from the baby is present, and it is only noticeably present when the baby's blood is being destroyed by Rh disease. In the event of significant sensitization, as evidenced by blood or amniotic fluid studies, the uterus is emptied by an induction or cesarean section—unless, of course, the pregnancy is too immature. Under these circumstances, we have developed a technique of transfusing the baby while it still lies within the uterus.

This technique is rarely used today, however, because there is now a vaccine that, given at the end of each pregnancy, counteracts the mother's Rh antibody production and so protects her next child. Since Rhogam has become available, Rh disease of the newborn has become exceedingly rare, and it is hoped that this disorder will eventually be completely within our control. The vaccine is given during the first few days following birth, after special tests performed upon the mother and baby determine that it is correct to do so. Rhogam is also given to Rh-negative women who abort spontaneously or who have a therapeutic abortion or an ectopic pregnancy. Moreover, it is now becoming popular to give the vaccine to Rh-negative women at about the 28th week of pregnancy, providing the Coombs' test is negative. This is an added protective factor for the mother and baby.

If you are a recently delivered Rh-negative mother—and you certainly should know your blood type—and no one is determining whether vaccine is indicated in your case during the first few postpartum days, be sure to bring the matter up with your doctor. Such a happenstance should never occur.

There are certain other rare types of isoimmunization (the term for blood incompatibility) from other unusual blood types. But, again, they are very rare and usually do not cause severe fetal problems.

Religion and Motherhood

Insofar as I can determine, there is no conflict between God and childbearing or childbirth. There are, however, certain conflictual situations that arise in pregnancy and childbirth as a result of our imperfect attempts to interpret God's word. This is not meant to offend anyone. Our religious leaders agree upon this "litany of imperfection." Our variety of faiths attests to it.

Now then, some of the very best hospitals in the world are Catholic. If I were in a strange community and sick, I would certainly go to a Catholic hospital without question. I would also go to a Jewish, Baptist, Lutheran, Presbyterian, or Methodist hospital with similar equanimity. Religious faith is not involved in my hospital decision; all the religious faiths that I am aware of run a tight ship and a good hospital.

The Catholic moral code, however, abuts rather sharply against some aspects of the management of pregnancy. In the first place, therapeutic abortion and sterilization by any means (unless the sterilization is incidental to some other procedure, say, a hysterectomy) are forbidden. But since both therapeutic abortion and sterilization are *elective* procedures, any sensible doctor would simply plan to perform them somewhere besides a Catholic hospital.

The most misunderstood article in the Catholic moral code states, in part, that you can't directly take a life to save another life. For generations the following misapplication of that doctrine has been widely circulated: If in, say, the conduct of labor, it becomes necessary to choose between saving a mother or her child, the child is saved and the mother allowed to die.

Now, I have practiced in a Catholic hospital for 25 years. During this time, we have delivered close to 100,000 mothers, and not once did this supposed conflict ever arise. During the same 25 years, eight expectant mothers died in that hospital, most of them from nonpregnancy causes (strokes, heart disease, embolism, and so forth). In no instance did anyone—or would anyone—have considered sacrificing a mother for *any* reason.

Maternal deaths must be reported. Hospital staff committees must investigate them. The worst thing an obstetrician can have on his record is a *preventable* maternal death. He must answer for his actions to his colleagues, not to the Catholic hospital.

Further, hospitals are inspected at least every two years by the Joint Commission of Hospital Accreditation (JCHA). Commission members are selected from the American Hospital Association, the American Medical Association, and the American College of Surgeons. Religion has nothing to do with the JCHA. This commission inspects every aspect of hospital care; it is incredibly meticulous and thorough. Its approval is *mandatory* for a hospital to function. One of the areas inspected most closely is the maternity division. Maternal and fetal death rates, infection rates, cesarean section rates, and many other statistics are studied. If a hospital, Catholic or not, in some way allowed a maternal death, supposedly to save an infant or for any other reason, the hospital would lose its accreditation. And so, without JCHA approval, that hospital could not have interns, residents, or nursing programs; it could not work with Medicare, Blue Cross, or any other health insurance carrier. Thus, accreditation is important—even vital—for a hospital's survival and function.

So you see that maternal deaths are studied closely by doctors and the JCHA in all hospitals, including Catholic ones, and therein lies the ultimate control of our level of practice.

Another area of religious involvement has to do with blood. At one time the leading cause of maternal death was hemorrhage. For a number of reasons, this is still mainly true, although total maternal deaths have vastly diminished. One factor has been the constant availability of blood in modern maternity units. Practitioners of some religious faiths, however, believe that blood transfusions are forbidden by God, even the auto-transfusion of a patient with her own spilled blood, a technically feasible procedure. Such limitations on hospitals and doctors are so restrictive that both will sometimes refuse to care for a patient who follows such a religion. A better solution, it appears, is for doctor and hospital to protect themselves as far as possible against legal assaults and then assume responsibility for that patient. I know, from personal experience, that it is a very arduous and sometimes frightening responsibility. But, in this bivouac of life, we are all God's children.

Alternative Medicine

A recent poll reveals that at least one-third of respondents had used at least one alternative medicine during the previous year. At least $1 billion are annually spent on such alternatives as natural medicines, acupuncture, homeotherapy, and other holistic practices. Some of these therapies are now covered by health plans.

I will not attempt to assess here the value of alternative treatments, but it is important to warn you about the impact of certain alternative situations on pregnancy.

- You should avoid any manipulations that tend to overextend your joints. As discussed in the section on exercise (pages 48–53), your joints are very sensitive to extension injury.

- While some "natural" medications probably have therapeutic benefits, it is also important to recognize that some are equally likely to produce dangerous and toxic reactions—just as some standard medications do. The difference is that there has been no standardization of these alternative medications, nor have studies been done of any toxic or teratogenic fetal effects they might have. It is judicious, then, to avoid them while you are pregnant. That only makes sense.

Proper Pregnant Pauses

- The first cesarean section performed in the United States was carried out by John Lambert Richmond in Newton, Ohio, in 1827. Two other doctors, Jesse Bennett of Virginia in 1794 and François Prevost in Donaldsville, Louisiana, in 1782, both claimed to have performed cesarean sections, but there is no adequate documentation of those claims. Richmond fully documented his procedure in the medical literature in 1830. The others did not, and the reports are hearsay. Both the mother and child involved in Doctor Richmond's operation survived!

- In an age when patient autonomy is considered paramount, forced cesarean interventions are a rarity—as they should be. But such events do continue to take place. The court may order such an intervention when, in the opinion of a medical ethics committee, it is justified. A physician presented with this problem—for example, an absolute pelvic disproportion and a mother refusing surgery— will involve the hospital ethics committee before going any further. If they agree with the doctor and the mother can still not be swayed, then a court order may be obtained and a forced section performed. A hospital's appropriate guidelines for proceeding with a forced section are further reinforced by the American College of Obstetricians and Gynecologists Committee on Ethics. This group makes every effort to protect the mother's rights while at the same time acknowledging the infant's rights. It is a sad and difficult journey.

•In 1975, 32 percent of mothers with children under the age of two were employed outside their homes. In 1996, that number had increased to 58 percent.

•The VBAC success rate is around 75 percent—depending upon the report one reads. About 50 percent of all mothers previously delivered by section should subsequently be able to deliver vaginally. How many are at this time being delivered by VBAC is not clearly known.

Diary

My Seventh Month

Problems_____

Medications_____

_____

_____

Rate of baby movement on a scale of 1–10_____

_____

Natural childbirth classes_____

_____

_____

Special tests_____

_____

_____

What's going on in the world?_____

_____

_____

_____

What's going on in my life?_____

_____

_____

_____

My thoughts and feelings_____

_____

_____

_____

Doctor's appointment_____

_____

_____

Questions to ask _____

_____

_____

_____

_____

_____

_____

_____

_____

_____

_____

_____

_____

_____

_____

_____

_____

_____

_____

_____

_____

_____

_____

_____

_____

_____

_____

_____

_____

_____

Eight

My Eighth Lunar Month

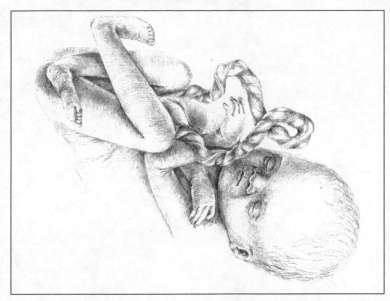

Now in its eighth lunar month, your infant is rapidly approaching maturity. By month's end it should weigh about four pounds (1,800 grams) and will measure 11.2 inches (28 centimeters). The skin is now well insulated with fat, there is usually plenty of scalp hair, and, if it is a young man within you, its testicles should now be in the scrotum.

There is no longer much room on this single ultrasound frame for more than the head. Again, the mouth is open as amniotic fluid is regularly being swallowed, and occasionally the fetus will grimace as if yawning. Intrauterine life may be boring!

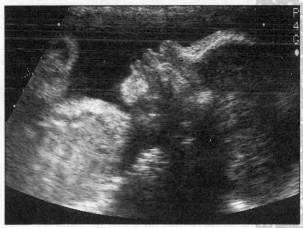

This point marks the beginning of your eighth lunar month—the 28th to 32nd weeks. During this time, your baby will be kicking actively in your throat, your side, and over your bladder, all at the same time, it seems. The reason you can feel movement in so many places simultaneously is that your baby is suspended, weightless, completely surrounded by water, like a skin diver, and it can move all four extremities at the same time. Also, your baby often has spontaneous rhythmic contractions of its diaphragm, which, for want of a better description, resemble hiccups. When you are lying still, you can feel these regular jerking movements. Your baby's skin is parchment-thin, and the blood vessels can be seen coursing through it in a very, very fine fan-like pattern. It can see and hear, but it doesn't really have very many chances to use these finely tuned capabilities. However, it now recognizes your voice. Born at the end of this month, a child has a 95 percent chance of survival and a 90 percent chance of survival free of major health prob-

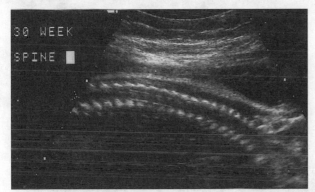

A close-up view of a 30-week fetal spine.

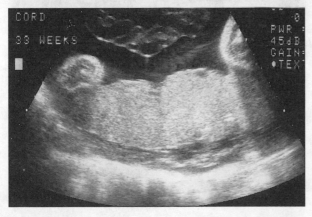

A segment of twisted umbilical cord coils can be seen in the upper portion of this ultrasound.

A fetal ear at 33 weeks.

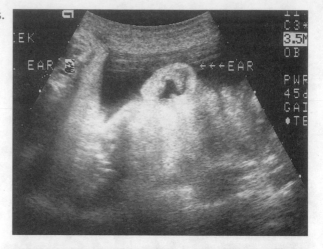

Looking directly down into a cross-section of a fetal heart at 32 weeks. The heart is the large black circle; it is bisected by two faint crosshairs representing the walls that divide it into four chambers—the normal anatomical configuration.

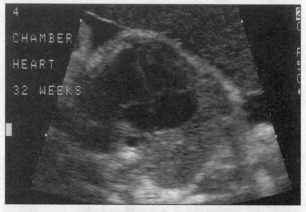

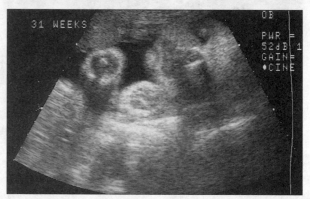

A fetal face at 31 weeks.

lems. The Dionne quintuplets were born at the beginning of this lunar month, and they all survived in a somewhat hostile environment. In their little home, there was no central heat, no electricity, and no running water or plumbing. Doctor Roy Allen Defoe, a venerable and true country doctor, kept them all alive by giving them, along with other nourishment, brandy and water in front of an open fireplace. Incubators were sent from Toronto to Corbiel—their birthplace in northern Ontario (where, incidentally, I was born), but with no electricity, the incubators could not be activated, nor oxygen flooded over them. Still, the little girls all survived—the first ever. While this book was being revised, we were blessed with an American birth of septuplets, who may well all survive. Moreover, we have had several surviving sets of quintuplets and one of sextuplets. These American multiple births, however, were all expected and planned for and took place in very friendly environments. None of these conditions greeted the Dionne quintuplets.

By the way, a few weeks ago you probably had a glucose challenge blood test, which I hope was within normal limits.

Premature Rupture of the Membranes (PROM)

Premature rupture of the membranes, a not uncommon obstetrical complication, occurs when the amniotic membranes that surround and enclose the infant break prior to the onset of labor—that is, prior to active, progressive dilation and thinning of the cervix. At or approaching full term, PROM does not create a very serious problem, since about 95 percent of the time spontaneous labor follows shortly thereafter. If it does not, the physician may resort to induction or, in some situations, cesarean section. Whatever the method used to effect labor and delivery, a mature child is what results, and we move on to the next problem—raising it!

On the other hand, PROM is a very serious problem when it involves a *preterm* pregnancy (now with its own acronym—pPROM). It puts both the expectant mother and her infant in significant jeopardy and is a many times more difficult and dangerous obstetrical problem to manage.

While PROM occurs in 10 percent of all pregnancies, only one in five of these are truly premature pregnancies (pPROM) as determined by fetal size and by dates. Regardless of what is done or not done in these cases, 70 percent will deliver within three days. Sometimes that is good, sometimes bad. Sometimes the baby is better off in the uterus, and sometimes it is better off in an incubator. It depends upon conditions in the mother or child that may be associated with the premature rupture. If, for instance, mother has severe preeclampsia and there is evidence of growth retardation, then the infant is better off in a neonatal unit.

Several situations cause pPROM, but it arises most commonly because of certain types of bacterial infection found at the back of the vagina—usually bacterial vaginosis, beta strep, or certain others (see the section on vaginal infections in chapter 4). When it does happen, any number of other events may follow—labor, abnormal presentation of the infant, infection (ainnionitis), cord prolapse, or respiratory distress syndrome in the infant (RDS).

Assessing the fetal status is the first step in managing early premature rupture of the membrane. Evidence of the degree of fetal maturity is sought by rechecking the clinical dates, doing repeated ultrasound examinations, and taking a transabdominal amniocentesis sample to determine fetal lung maturity. Further assessment of the fetus would include observation and studies for potential infection—particularly the potential of spread from the vaginal infection below. Such factors as maternal fever, increased fetal heart rate, and amniotic fluid abnormalities might indicate active or incipient infection.

Once the physician determines the fetal status, he or she must decide whether to effect delivery at once. If delivery is not indicated, there are numerous ways of attempting to prevent premature labor, as you will see in the next section. However, with pPROM in the presence of infection or certain other complications, it is not wise to halt labor. In fact, as mentioned earlier, it may be better to have the child delivered and in a safer environment—a neonatal intensive-care unit.

Sometimes cortisone and other steroid agents are given during the latent period before labor begins or is initiated, to try to increase the maturity of the infant's lungs, and antibiotics are given to try to arrest infection. Deciding whether to use these agents requires a great deal of skill and judgment, and each case must be treated individually.

As always, what has been said here is a broad general outline of the problem and the various modes of treatment. Again, your own doctor will know the best way to proceed if this complication should appear in your pregnancy.

Prematurity and Premature Labor

About one of every 10–12 pregnancies ends prematurely. Prematurity is thus a vastly important area of obstetrics, since it can cause significant fetal and newborn problems. Believe it or not, premature birth is one of the leading causes of all American mortality. Add to this the complications of managing our premature survivors and you begin to become aware of the magnitude of our responsibilities toward the prematurely born.

First of all, what is considered a premature birth? Well, in terms of size, an infant whose weight at birth is 5 pounds, 8 ounces (2,500 grams) or less is deemed premature. In terms of time, any child born before the 37th week is considered premature. Neither statistical guideline is entirely satisfactory; as we saw in the section on intrauterine growth retardation in chapter 6, any child born early or small and, as a result, unable to cope with life outside the uterus may be called premature. We also note that in some countries ethnic differences result in smaller babies because of genetic constitution. Therefore, it is difficult to make any worthwhile comparisons of survival or treatment between different ethnic groups and countries.

The causes of premature labor are diverse. Many of them are interrelated and many are not. In the first place, we as doctors create a certain amount of prematurity when we induce labor in the threatening medical conditions already noted elsewhere in the book. Thus, hypertension of pregnancy, IUGR, diabetes, Rh disorders, and so on may lead us to empty the uterus early, since the fetus is no longer safe within it. We have also contributed to prematurity by doing repeat elective cesarean sections prior to full maturity. These unfortunate events have occurred in the best regulated practices but are now a very minor contribution to prematurity.

Having put those factors aside, let us look at the most common causes of prematurity:

- malnutrition

- a very young or very old mother

- premature rupture of the membranes associated with vaginal infection

- tobacco, alcohol, or drug use

- maternal chronic disease—diabetes, hypertension, renal disorders, and so on

- maternal acute illness—fever, acute pyelitis, and so on

- abnormal uterine size or shape, such as is found in the presence of tumors or congenital malformation

- multiple pregnancy

- weakness of the cervix (incompetent cervical os)

- incompetent cervical problems treated by surgical closure

- abnormal placental location or premature separation of the placenta

- cervical surgery such as conization for precancer

- excess amniotic fluid (polyhydramnios)

- two previous second-trimester abortions

What are the problems that prematurity brings to the little ones? Well, it's like a blastoff before the astronaut has put on his space suit, buckled down, and attached his oxygen line. The worst problem is usually that the newborn's lungs aren't ready to breathe; in addition, its temperature-control mechanism is weak, and its digestive, excretory, and enzyme systems are not all quite "go." It doesn't have sufficient fat deposits to insulate against temperature changes. But blastoff has come and gone, so what do we do?

First, labor must be managed most carefully; pain relief measures should be those least likely to depress the baby. Monitoring of fetal activity and well-being should be continued throughout labor and delivery. Following delivery, the infant should be immediately transferred to an intensive-care nursery. This is the best environment in which to minimize the effects of respiratory distress syndrome (RDS), the most likely opponent of the baby's well-being, and to cope with the other critical problems that may arise.

Dramatic improvement in the survival rate of small prematures is now the order of the day, as is the quality of their survival—as we have seen. A baby weighing less than one pound has already survived in the intensive neonatal care environment—and is healthy today. Such success is due to modern intensive-care nurseries, the marvelous nurses staffing them, neonatologists, and very highly skilled pediatricians.

Prevention of premature labor is the best solution for all these problems. However, this is very difficult to achieve, since success depends upon the control of so many variables. Looking at the list of causes of premature labor, it is clear that some factors can be controlled. Close management of systemic diseases, diet supplementation, the avoidance of drugs, appropriate adolescent sexual counseling, the early treatment of vaginal infections—these therapies will all make a difference.

Still, premature labor will take place, and being able to detect it early on is important in trying to arrest it. It is very helpful, therefore, to be able to discover those pregnancies destined to premature labor before the event is upon us. To achieve this goal, we have set in place a series of procedures.

- •Women at risk for premature labor are watched for the following potentially **indicative signs:**
  - constant low-back pain
  - frequent abdominal tightening
  - menstrual-like cramps
  - pelvic pressure
  - spotting or a marked increase in mucoid discharge

- •**Home uterine monitoring.** Equipment is available for monitoring uterine contractions at home. An abdominal transducer is worn at regular intervals and the uterine contraction patterns recorded by the mother or transmitted via phone lines to her obstetrician's office. The absolute value of this procedure has not been clearly proven as yet, but it would appear to be a step forward.

- Predicting premature labor with some sort of **test or procedure** has always been one of our goals. These goals are gradually being achieved.

- **Ultrasound determinations of the cervical length** as pregnancy advances have become very accurate—so much so that measurements of this length have become a guideline for determining the onset of premature labor—the longer the cervix, the better.

- A variety of new **biochemical tests** also have a certain potential for establishing premature labor risk. They include levels of fetal fibronectin, elevated interleukin–6 amniotic values, and maternal salivary estriol content. Each of these procedures has its detractors and its supporters, and as our experience grows, each becomes a better marker of premature labor risk. They all have value.

Once premature labor has become established, several tocolytic (labor-arresting) interventions are commonly employed to delay labor—if only long enough to gain more fetal maturity (even seven days makes a significant difference) and administer cortisone, which, crossing the placenta and gaining access to the infant, will mature its lungs very rapidly and thus help avoid respiratory distress syndrome.

Labor-arresting interventions fall into the following chemical categories:

- **Ritodrine.** This chemical is FDA-approved for use in the control of premature labor. It is a very powerful and potentially dangerous drug that must be used only in institutions quite capable of handling it as well as certain potential complications to the mother, particularly her cardiovascular system. Generally it is administered intravenously at the beginning of premature labor; if successful and safe, the oral route is used for long-term treatment, both in the hospital and at home.

- **Magnesium sulfate.** Traditionally this chemical has been used—and indeed is still used—for the control of hypertension of pregnancy. But it is also a uterine muscle relaxant, and so it is used to prevent premature labor, particularly in those patients for whom Ritodrine would be unsafe. Magnesium sulfate is administered intravenously at the beginning of treatment, and, if successful, the mode of administration may be switched at a later time.

•**Terbutaline.** Another uterine relaxant in the Ritodrine family, its risks and benefits are about the same.

Certain other agents are now being used on an experimental basis only and have no place yet in general tocolysis programs.

Again, these drugs are exceedingly active and may have profound effects upon the expectant mother and the fetus. They must be used judiciously according to strict protocols. But first you and your doctor must carefully weigh the benefits and risks of whichever agent is chosen.

Perinatology

This specialty (also called perinatal medicine and, more recently, maternal-fetal medicine) has become an obstetrical subspecialty. These highly trained obstetricians deal entirely with very complicated maternity problems. Their training includes the management of significant maternal medical and obstetrical complications and the impact of these problems on the fetus. Perinatologists practice almost exclusively in class III maternity units (see page 301), which provide adequate facilities for carrying out their special care. In this environment, the perinatologist studies maternal health, nutrition, and body functions, particularly in high-risk mothers. Using electronic and laboratory monitoring, he or she observes the growth and development of the baby, gauges placental reserve, and, finally, intensively monitors both mother and child during labor and delivery, with all the equipment and judgment available in today's superb health care system.

Neonatology

The neonatologist is a highly specialized pediatrician who takes care of endangered newborns in an intensive-care nursery—which, incidentally, resembles the flight deck of a spaceship. There are instruments to measure everything and to feed, breathe for, and heat—everything except fondle—sick newborns until they can make it on their own. Very premature babies, those born of high-risk mothers, babies who have gone through a difficult labor or delivery, babies stressed from any cause whatsoever—all can enter the intensive-care environment and be ministered to with the specialized skills of a neonatologist, accompanied by a skilled nursing staff, and stand an excellent chance of undamaged survival.

Metabolic Changes in Late Pregnancy

During these last few months, your basal metabolic rate—the rate at which fuel (carbohydrates) is burned by oxygen in your body—increases. This rise persists until your delivery, at which time it drops very rapidly to slightly below normal, where it stays for several months. These changes in metabolism cause you to have more energy during late pregnancy, but they also decrease your tolerance of heat and your ability to sleep. If your last trimester happens to fall in the summertime, you can be very uncomfortable indeed. Insomnia, for this and many other reasons, is even more common now, and sleep becomes a precious commodity. Turn up the air conditioner and get a two-foot-wide blanket for your husband.

Pain Again

Numerous localities in your anatomy may now begin to ache, puff, crack, turn up, turn down, turn out, bend, swell, hurt, sag, explode, get numb, and get sore—not in any serious way at all, but just enough to let you know that your passenger is demanding more space all the time and so something's got to give. And it's you!

Rib Pain

For one thing, your passenger is pushing everything that used to be in your lower abdomen into your upper abdomen, and everything that was in your upper abdomen into your chest. As a result, your rib cage has to expand, the lower ribs frequently separating spontaneously from the breastbone (sternum). These free-floating ribs can produce considerable local discomfort, particularly on your right side—the side that also must accommodate your liver. The discomfort continues off and on until you have delivered, at which time the rib cage closes again and the separated members rejoin the breastbone. Like so many of the lesser burdens you have to bear at this time, nothing can be done to prevent or correct rib separation. Everything has got to go somewhere.

Pressure Pain

At the other end of the line, your precious passenger packs the bladder, the rectum, and all the pelvic organs into a wafer-like compress. This crowding produces a significant amount of lower abdominal discomfort, bladder and rectal pressure, pressure transmitted into the back, down the legs, and so on. Sometimes it is helpful to wear a supportive maternity girdle, which raises the infant out of your lower abdomen. Generally, however, it just pushes the load further under your ribs, with predictable results up above. Not to worry—no damage is being done.

Braxton-Hicks Contractions

During the third month of pregnancy, your uterus begins to contract rhythmically in order to help circulate blood through it. The contractions continue throughout pregnancy and are usually painless. You may tell your doctor that the baby is knotting up in your abdomen, though it is not the baby but the muscles of the uterus that produce the sensation. (This same knotting occurs during labor, but then, because of certain differences in what is going on, discomfort is produced.) Occasionally these early contractions, named after the obstetrician who first described them (but never felt them), are painful, and occasionally they produce false labor. There is no danger that Braxton-Hicks contractions, even though painful, will produce real labor. When they annoy you too much, lie down and try to relax. Read in chapter 10 how you can identify false labor and differentiate it from the real thing. A warning, though: If you are a candidate for premature labor for any of the reasons mentioned earlier, or if your doctor feels that you may be a candidate, painful uterine contractions must not be ignored. Even intense painless contractions may be a signal to call in.

Numb Spots

Although numbness cannot generally be equated with pain, it is still an unpleasant sensation, and pregnancy produces its own little points of numbness. One popular area is the abdomen, which, as it expands, stretches the superficial nerve fibers that spread out to cover the skin. As a result, certain areas in the upper abdomen and over the lower rib cage often become numb and occasionally become exquisitely sensitive to touch, including the rub of clothing.

Likewise, it is not uncommon to have numbness and tingling in your fingers in the last few months of pregnancy. This is produced by swelling of the supportive tissue tunnels that carry the major nerve trunks into the arms and hands. The condition is called carpal tunnel syndrome. Diuretics (water pills) sometimes reduce the swelling in these tissue tunnels, but they are not very successful and certainly are not to be recommended during pregnancy just to manage that problem. Although no permanent damage has been clearly demonstrated by carpal tunnel syndrome during pregnancy, it has occurred in certain other medical situations in which some nerve disability has followed, and so it would be well for you to at least advise your doctor of this sensation. Sometimes, if the swelling occurs in higher nerve tunnels, relief may be obtained by sleeping with a figure-of-eight Ace bandage woven across the shoulders. Try it!

Umbilical Hernia

Most of us have a little defect in the abdominal wall around the area of our navels (the umbilicus). This is the exact spot where your connection to your own mother entered your body in bygone days. During pregnancy, your inside abdominal pressure may become sufficient for that defect to open slightly and some of your intestines may protrude into it—so, suddenly, you have an umbilical hernia. You will see and feel a little bulge around your navel which may be slightly tender. Usually you can painlessly push (reduce) the hernia back in with your finger; you may want to keep it in with a piece of cotton taped over it. Very rarely, the hernia gets trapped in its new little compartment. If it should get seriously trapped, you would know it by the significant pain it produces, and you would need—you would want—to call for help post-haste. Of course, after delivery, like everything else, these little sacs generally disappear.

Occasionally, your belly button just everts, owing to the internal pressure, but there is nothing in it.

These little aches and pains, then, generally have no temporary or permanent consequences, but they do occur and may cause you to wonder a bit about what is going on. There may be some other little area skirmishes that I have not covered here, or elsewhere; if so, please let me know.

Breast-Feeding

It is very clear that most of us physicians know little about the physiology and mechanics of breast-feeding and therefore offer poor support to women interested in this most rewarding endeavor. A recent study reveals that, although 60 percent of all mothers left the hospital nursing their babes, within a few weeks the numbers began dwindling, and by six months, only 20 percent continued to nurse. Other studies reveal that only 45 percent of all obstetricians and pediatricians encouraged mothers to breast-feed. Moreover, most medical students and hospital resident physicians agreed that they were inadequately trained in counseling mothers about breast-feeding. So the profession has not been geared to manage this responsibility—so much so that a group of physicians have recently initiated a very important and promising endeavor: forming the Academy of Breast-feeding Medicine in order to spread the message to us all.

There are certainly problems getting started with nursing, but if mothers are prepared for it, and their initial problems are managed properly, continued nursing becomes a fulfilling, healthy bonding experience for both mother and child. Breast-feeding is a natural resource of compound importance and should be promoted by everyone involved in maternity care. To this end, the U.S. Public Health Service has set a goal for the year 2000—to have 75 percent of all mothers initiate breast-feeding, with 50 percent continuing it. This is a very worthwhile goal, but we do not appear to be on target at the moment.

Let's look at some of the advantages of breast-feeding—advantages for both mother and child.

- •For the mother:
  reduced postpartum blood loss
  reduced risk of later ovarian or breast cancer
  birth control
  no formula problems

- •For the infant:
  immunity instantly provided against many infections during the
    early weeks after birth
  a decreased incidence of diarrhea, otitis media (ear infection),
    lower respiratory tract infection, and bacterial meningitis
  protection against sudden infant death syndrome (SIDS), insulin-
    dependent diabetes mellitus, ulcerative colitis, and Crohn's
    disease

It is also worth mentioning the personal cost savings and the solid-waste savings of billions of plastic containers.

There are two early problems associated with nursing that often discourage beginning mothers.

- •**Sore nipples.** Even when nipples are properly prepared all along for nursing by gentle lanolin or other skin cream massage and equally gentle eversion stripping, nipple tenderness may still develop early on. It is important that whoever is helping you manage breast-feeding be made aware of this problem. It can often be overcome by ensuring that you are using the proper nursing position. When the baby cannot latch on properly because of nursing position, its suckling action will surely cause nipple soreness. Improper positioning may also prevent the infant from obtaining all the milk that is available. Moreover, when the baby suckles only on the nipple and not the surrounding areola, there is more likely to be nipple tenderness. When these problems are overcome, nipple tenderness usually disappears.

•**Perceived low milk supply.** The perception that the infant is not getting enough milk because not enough is being made leads to a self-fulfilling defeat. Supplementation leads to less breast stimulation, and therefore less milk. Moreover, suckling on a bottle teaches the infant new suckling responses that will not work on the breast, thus further diminishing the chance of successful nursing. Babies are born with adequate food stores to keep them going in the early days.

Breasts do become very engorged and tender shortly after delivery. This phenomenon, however, is not milk coming in but rather the priming of breast glands in order to get started. When engorgement fades away but a ton of milk is not yet flowing, the priming is only just beginning to work.

To nurse is to complete the natural human cycle of pregnancy, delivery, and child-rearing. If it is your wish, and if you are able, nursing is of great psychological benefit to both you and your child and you should do it. On the other hand, if it is not your wish to nurse, and you do so because of outside pressure or because you feel you should, breast-feeding will become a burden surrounded by tension, apprehension, and disenchantment. Your baby will very rapidly sense this, and the result will be more harm than good to your relationship. You yourself should decide whether to nurse after reviewing the available information and assessing your own wishes, values, and desires.

Here is a list of information about the pros and cons of breast-feeding:

•Breast-feeding is not advisable when the mother is a hepatitis B carrier, if she is severely ill with a systemic disorder, or if she is markedly anemic. It may also not be recommended if she has active toxoplasmosis or cytomegalovirus, is on hard drugs or dangerous medication, or smokes excessively.

•More bottle-fed infants die in epidemics of gastroenteritis than do breast-fed babies.

•Human milk contains a substance, lactoferrin, that inhibits the growth of certain pathological bacteria in the intestines.

•Breast-fed babies have fewer allergies and never have calcium-deficiency muscle spasms.

•Cow's milk contains more sodium and chloride than does human milk. This may produce dehydration, particularly if solid foods are introduced too early.

•Human milk contains a substance that triggers the baby's appetite control mechanism. The breast-fed baby is thus less likely to be an obese baby. Obese babies become obese adults.

- Animal milk may become contaminated if sterile precautions are not observed. Human milk may be contaminated only as noted in the first item of this list.

- Breast-feeding, if enjoyed, is psychologically better than bottle-feeding for both participants.

- Physicians very seldom use hormones after delivery to suppress lactation. Certain medications are given to mothers who cannot or will not nurse, but generally they are not hormone substances, and they must usually be taken for a fairly long time.

- Although young nursing mothers take somewhat longer to shed pounds, new research indicates that fairly rapid weight loss programs, if they are nutritious and include plenty of fluids, will not disturb breast-feeding.

- Nursing mothers lose calcium from their bones which cannot be replaced even by adequate calcium intake. This is probably due to the temporary suppression of estrogen production by nursing—much like what takes place in the menopause. This loss, however, is temporary, and calcium is soon replaced when estrogen production returns.

Here follows a modified list of breast-feeding basics prepared by Herbert Goldenring, an associate clinical professor at Yale University.

- Every full-term healthy newborn has a built-in 2–3-day food supply. Colostrum, the lemony yellow first milk, contains the immunity factors that protect the baby for up to six weeks. Colostrum can be considered the baby's first immunity—which only the mother can provide.

- A large volume of breast milk does not come in for three or four days and depends upon the frequency of the baby's suckling as well as the mother's hormonal response.

- Every baby is different! Some come out as "barracudas" and eat like a veteran from the start. Others may be "connoisseurs" and take two or three sucks, stop a while, then return for a few more. Anything in between is possible.

- After feeding, mothers will become very thirsty and should drink eight ounces of clear fluids at the end of each session. This practice will also help prevent constipation.

- The baby should suck not only on the nipple but on the surrounding areola. The correct latch-on position for the baby is very important.

•The baby empties the breast in six to eight minutes. The highest fat content is in the last portion of each feeding. Feedings should allow ten minutes on one breast, then burp (the baby), then ten to fifteen minutes on the other.

•Until the milk comes in, feed every three hours, or more frequently if the baby is fussy. Once the milk is in, feedings should be every two to four hours. It takes about two hours to develop an adequate milk supply. After about four hours, gently wake the baby during the day and feed. This may prevent the baby from turning day into night.

•When the milk comes in, there may be more than the baby needs. This is a good time to pump the breasts and store some in the freezer. At two to four weeks, the baby will feed more frequently for a few days. This may also occur at six to eight weeks and much later at about six months.

•If the baby wets six to eight diapers a day, he or she is getting enough milk.

For more information on breast-feeding:

•Contact your local La Leche League, which is in the telephone book.

•Read *A Practical Guide to Breast-feeding* by Jan Riordan (Boston: Jones and Bartlett, June 1996).

Milk

Mention has been made before about the good and the bad in cow's milk; let's bring all this information together here.

Normally infants produce enough lactase until age two to handle all the milk they can get—from mother or wherever. Thereafter, lactase levels drop rapidly. Lactase is the enzyme that digests milk sugar—lactose. It is safe to say, then, that milk, particularly human milk, is good baby food. After two years of age, people and milk should probably begin to part company. Here's why:

•About 50 million Americans (one in four) cannot tolerate lactose (milk sugar) because of low lactase levels in their bodies. Milk gives these adults and older children cramps, bloating, fullness, and occasionally diarrhea. Further, if milk in any quantity is consumed, lactose intolerance can interfere with carbohydrate and, possibly, protein metabolism.

• True milk allergy occurs in up to 7 percent of the population; for them, the ingestion of milk produces allergic reactions of various kinds and severity.

• Yogurt—milk that is naturally fermented with lactobacillus—has had most of its lactose inactivated or hydrolyzed. It is therefore safe food for lactose-intolerant and milk-allergic people. However, most commercial yogurt is not so prepared. Read the label. Yogurt should be low-fat or fat-free.

• Adults should restrict milk intake to one pint of skim milk a day because milk—particularly whole milk, and more particularly homogenized milk—is rich in cholesterol, a prime mover in heart disease.

• Pregnant women (and newborn babies) who drink cow's milk can have calcium-deficiency muscle spasms. Calcium absorption from cow's milk is blocked by other substances in it. We have already seen that newborns on mother's milk do not have this problem. Expectant mothers experience these muscle symptoms in the form of early-morning leg cramps.

• There is now mounting evidence that the introduction of cow's milk into human diets is a primary cause of insulin-dependent diabetes mellitus. The diabetic tendency in humans may be compared to a loaded gun waiting for some force to pull the trigger. That force is usually a foreign protein, and several research studies have identified that foreign protein as cow's milk. Visible clinical evidence of diabetes may take years to appear, but the gun has been fired.

Standard pregnancy diets (but not the one recommended in this book) have traditionally included at least one quart of cow's milk daily. Studies show that lactose-intolerant pregnant women (one in four, remember) who are forced to consume at least one quart of milk daily have significantly smaller babies than pregnant women who do not drink milk.

The Placenta

This piece of biological equipment, commonly called the afterbirth, is made by your baby and belongs to your baby. It connects you to each other by partially invading the inner surface of your uterus. Why you don't reject it (since it is an organ transplant from another human being) and why it stops invading your body at the very point it does, have been the subjects of much study and considerable theorizing. Very rarely, the placenta goes wild and invades its host (you), causing what was once the most fatal of all cancers. Fortunately, it is now a very curable cancer.

At full term, a placenta is a bloody, spongy, pie-shaped organ weighing about two pounds, with membranes trailing off its edges. It has a life span of about nine months. The placenta dies, of course, at birth, and under the microscope it shows all the signs of old age—including hardening of the arteries.

There is tremendous "reserve" in normal placentas. This reserve protects the baby if the placenta becomes partially detached or if placental senescence (premature aging) robs the fetus of necessary food and oxygen, thus producing distress.

Your baby's heart pumps its blood back and forth through the umbilical cord and into the placenta. It never normally comes directly in touch with your blood but, as in a heart-lung machine, is always separated by a membrane of sorts. It is true, however, as you have seen with the Rh disorders, that small spurts of fetal blood can escape into the maternal circulation, particularly in late pregnancy, but these are very minor connections indeed. Bathing on one side of this membrane, your baby's blood pulls food and oxygen over from you—plus alcohol, nicotine, medicine, drugs, or whatever else happens to be floating past at the time. In return, the baby slips you carbon dioxide and other waste products for you to eliminate. So you are eating for two and excreting for two—though, of course, one of you two is a very small user and dumper!

The placenta secretes a number of hormones that trigger all sorts of responses, both locally and around your body. Mainly it produces chorionic gonadotropin (which, you remember, makes pregnancy tests positive, breasts grow, menstruation stop, and so on), progesterone (which allows the uterus to grow and not expel the baby until the time comes), and certain other hormones and enzymes, some of which can have powerful systemic effects on your blood pressure, metabolism, breasts, lactation, and so on.

New discoveries of substances called prostaglandins, along with the corticotropin-releasing hormones (CRH) circulating throughout our bodies, have yielded information about the onset of labor. The placenta, it appears, is programmed to secrete certain prostaglandins and CRH in large amounts during its dying days. These substances can overcome all uterine relaxants and protectants, and so labor begins. But it is not really quite that simple. Other programs are certainly involved in the onset of labor.

Most placentas are discarded at birth, but occasionally one ends up in the laboratory if it appears unusual in any important way or is needed as part of a specific research program. Moreover, some pharmaceutical companies in the United States buy placentas and use them in order to extract certain very specific and powerful hormones, which they use either in research or in hormone manufacturing. They don't pay very much for the used placentas, so don't expect a cut in your hospital bill!

You may have heard that cord (and placental) blood is now being collected and stored in a frozen state for future therapeutic uses in the treatment of cancer. See the appendix for a complete discussion of this program.

Newborn Insurance

Practically all 50 states now have legislation that requires all family health insurance policies to cover newborns from the moment of birth. Until recently, most family insurance policies were written to cover the costs for treatment of newborn illness or defects, but some did not cover the first 14–30 days. The new laws cover any baby for any illness or complication needing treatment from the moment he or she is born.

Contact your insurance agent and make sure your policy covers newborns. To make this part of your policy effective, you must notify your insurance carrier within 30 days of your baby's birth, providing baby's birth date, name, sex, and parents' insurance policy number.

Managed care programs (HMOs, PPOs, and so on) have recently made vast inroads in this area, and it is therefore very important that you be aware of the protection provided—or not provided—by these companies. Call yours—maybe you can get through to a humanoid!

Preparation for Childbirth

First, about pain. Recently there appeared a fascinating newspaper column by a very well known and highly respected writer. Her thesis was that the millions of women who conceive each year against their wishes, simply because they failed to use simple, readily available birth control methods, are *stupid*. She herself is a liberated American woman (what Rush Limbaugh likes to call a "Feminazi"!) who speaks freely, fiercely, and regularly on these matters. She is highly regarded by many other women. I wonder, however, what would happen to me had I written the same column. Probably the same fate that would befall someone making a third-party entrance into a husband-wife quarrel!

And so it is that a man has some meaningful hesitation—if he has any sense—before making any remarks concerning pain in childbearing. I have participated (as much as possible) in many thousands of deliveries, both before and after preparedness, before and after "deep sleep" (also called "twilight"—a program now in its own twilight), and before and after epidurals; I have delivered babies in hospitals, homes, taxis, airplanes, trains, bathrooms—you name it. I thus at least have a feeling for the subject I am about to skirt around.

It is best to avoid the term *natural childbirth,* coined by Dr. Grantly Dick Read in his original work on preparation for childbearing. "Natural childbirth" denotes what took place in all the millennia prior to the scientific era of obstetrics—which at least began early in this century when medicine was primitive and dress was elegant. (Now the reverse is true!) In those early times, many women conceived and delivered without difficulty. Because of natural selection, the weak and deformed babies died before or at birth, and expectant mothers who had any severe obstetrical problem or complication, no matter how strong they may have been, often went with their babies. This was, and still is, the law of nature in every other species; being nature's way, it is truly "natural childbirth." Family plots in old cemeteries bear eloquent silent witness to that fact.

It is also very true that when we physicians began assisting in the birthing chamber, we committed many errors, and many women and their children suffered while doctors were learning the specialized knowledge so long denied. However, as a result of these pioneer efforts, a high level of safety for mother and child has finally been achieved—to the point that some of us, with a false sense of security generated by hospital and birthing center safety, have chosen to separate and deliver far from this unnatural environment that we have created. But more on this later. We must get back to pain.

There is no "curse of Eve." Women were not, and are not, destined or ordained to bring forth children in pain and sorrow. Adam didn't have to eat that apple.

Even disregarding very abnormal obstructed labor, pain-producing events occur during normal labor. If, however, not all pain sensation is perceived by the laboring mother, then a block must have arisen from within—a block produced by endorphins, which are always present but may be heightened by, and related to, enlightenment or preparation. The same effect can sometimes be achieved by placebos and by other sensory stimuli such as hypnosis. Endorphins can also be strongly stimulated by prayer.

Doctors did not introduce pain in childbearing—it was there when they arrived. One does not have to rely on history to confirm that fact—there are plenty of areas in our world today where that observation may still be confirmed. The doctor's role has not been to make pain and instill fear, but to release laboring women from such burdens. And so they did, starting in a society that was not ready to accept anything but some kind of sedation—whiskey, as often as not. There was great apprehension about what would happen to women—what might be done to them—as they slept their pain away. Queen Victoria made a giant step forward for us by demanding ether for the delivery of Prince Edward.

And so it was, after all, doctors who, released from the constant combat with death and disability in the early delivery chambers, first developed the concept of mature preparedness for childbirth and thus released patients from the heavy sedation that had helped them gain their foothold. Regular obstetricians may have been slow in accepting the newer concepts, but *so were their patients*. Thus, doctors who moved forward too fast left their patients behind and soon had no practice at all.

The introduction, then, of advanced programs for the prepared childbirth experience marked a giant step forward in obstetrical care. Not only did it reduce and sometimes obliterate the need for excessive sedation and depressant medications during labor, it further enhanced the whole birthing experience for everyone involved—mother, father, siblings, and attendants.

The modern era of prepared childbirth, then, began in the 1950s with the publication of Dr. Grantly Dick Read's work on "natural" childbirth, *Childbirth Without Fear*. He believed that bearing and delivering a child is a normal physiological event, and that with proper preparation and knowledge, and with the absence of fear, pain could be considerably reduced.

The Read fervor gradually dissipated, however, and various other prepared childbirth programs became more popular. At the same time, classes for expectant parents and training exercises continued. Today the Lamaze program, with its many and varied modifications, has become far and away the most popular approach to planned labor and delivery. Fundamentally, Dr. Lamaze felt that women should be prepared emotionally and psychologically for childbirth in accordance with Pavlov's principle of conditioned responses. According to this principle, which has been called psychoprophylaxis, the brain can be trained to accept any given stimulus and to select its response. Lamaze believed that laboring women could be trained to respond in a positive fashion to the contractions of their uterus during labor and delivery, and also to the attendant stretching of the tissues throughout the birth canal and vagina at the time of delivery.

The American Lamaze method differs from the French and Russian versions, and indeed, there are as many varieties of this approach to conditioning for labor as there are teachers. The basic philosophy, however, remains unchanged. It is not necessarily childbirth without pain, nor is it necessarily childbirth without anesthesia; it is positive conditioning used as training for the birth experience.

Education for childbirth is a magnificent concept *when it remains factual*. Knowledge diminishes fear and increases cooperation. The need for—indeed, the desire for—drugs is diminished. Childbirth becomes a joyful experience, and I heartily recommend it to you. Educated childbirth is not natural childbirth, however, since it requires learning procedures and techniques that not only alter the environment but are impossible for some women to master.

The need for anesthetic support in any type of prepared delivery should not be regarded as a failure of the technique or of the mother; nor should it be attended by any sense of shame or guilt by the mother, or fear for her child's safety or health. One of the sad disadvantages of any of these techniques is that the pregnant woman may have learned at the feet of an overzealous teacher who believes and teaches that everyone should, must, can win the gold. This attitude produces a sense of failure and shame among the other medalists. All you need to do is your very best in a warm supportive environment.

When both prospective participants are in agreement, it is altogether desirable for a husband, live-in mate, or close friend to participate in the labor and delivery process and, indeed, in the classes. Only then should it be done. Some partners, however, get see-sick and frightened. Moreover, some men find that the degree of intimacy involved in sharing this fundamental experience with their partner is more than they can reasonably and positively deal with. Consequently, for them the affair is neither fulfilling nor rewarding and does nothing to increase their ability to be intimate in the future. Indeed, for some the reverse is true: Particularly when participation is forced upon them by peer or other pressures, they may become more detached, with long-term negative psychological consequences for the relationship. The choice of whether to be present in the delivery room is a highly personal one, best left to the individual.

Altered Hospital Settings

The strict hospital rules that once isolated laboring women from their families and friends were instituted by physicians generations ago to reduce the risk of infection and for a number of other reasons that no longer exist. To pry us out of this long-casted mold required a good deal of consumer pressure, but opening up the delivery room turned out to be an altogether good and rewarding change. Women had been denied preparation for childbirth, a warm laboring environment, and the company of their loved ones during labor. They eventually revolted and started moving back toward home deliveries. This movement has gained momentum over the past decade, and while it is an altogether pleasant way to have a normal delivery, home birthing can be truly dangerous—as past history reveals to us. But let's have a look at the effect that the home birth movement has had upon our hospital environment.

In most hospitals now offering obstetrical care, birthing rooms and modified delivery rooms are now in place. In a typical birthing room, the furnishings are those of an average bedroom, with most of the obstetrical equipment blocked from view by a variety of mechanisms. In such a setting, women may labor in a home-like environment, with their family and friends present, as their wishes dictate, and in a bed that can be taken apart during the time of delivery so that the doctor has easy access to carry out the delivery procedures. In the event that some unforeseen complication develops, all the facilities that the hospital can marshal are readily available, either in a sectioned-off area of the bedroom or in a nearby delivery suite. All the hospital laboratory facilities and anesthesia capabilities are also close by. Many times it is possible to labor and deliver in a birthing room and then be allowed to go home a few hours after delivery without ever having been formally admitted to the hospital. But there are great advantages to just being there.

Separate birthing facilities with close hospital ties are also taking hold in some communities. Moreover, trained and competent midwives—usually working in company with an obstetrician or a group of them—are now managing normal obstetrical cases with great success.

In all these altered situations, there is a chain of responsibility that can quickly move a mother with a birthing problem into the appropriate setting for her particular care.

And finally, hospitals are now sponsoring not only prepared childbirth classes but parenting, sibling, and nursing classes that involve the family as a unit. They have almost always met with great acceptance by the community *and* the medical profession.

Prepared Pregnant Pauses

- There are approximately 177 million births throughout the world each year, and 500,000 maternal deaths (300 per 100,000 live births). There are approximately 3,913,000 births in the United States each year, and, most recently, 277 maternal deaths (7.1 per 100,000 live births).

- In 1996, there were 5,847 female deaths from firearms, and in some areas of our country, death from firearms was the *leading* cause of maternal mortality! And just to keep things in further perspective, over 300 women were killed in 1996 when they were struck by an automobile while bicycling!

•A recent study by a group of psychologists shows that the risk of premature delivery was doubled for both white and black women when a positive pregnancy anticipation was combined with high or rising levels of stress. Conversely, both groups experienced a slight decrease in premature labor despite an anxiety-producing lifestyle if there also existed a low pregnancy desirability. Figure that out!

•The fetus within you can hear what goes on outside, so you may want to watch your language. There is ample evidence that the fetus comes to know your voice and recognizes it at the time of birth. That's why he or she may turn to you when placed on your abdomen following delivery. It is also becoming clear that a child's behavioral patterns and characteristic traits are exhibited in the uterus from about the 28th week on and may become well enough established to predict some characteristics of the newborn.

•United Nations health workers in a Third World country recently received a directive warning them that both sexes should be immunized simultaneously in any preventive health program. This directive was issued because a previous group of workers began inoculating just the women of a certain tribe with tetanus vaccine. The men mistakenly assumed that their women were getting shots of long-acting birth control medication. Thus followed a rash of pregnancies!

•The American College of Obstetricians and Gynecologists has long recommended that women be provided at least 14 prenatal office visits as a part of normal pregnancy care. However, a study recently published in the *Journal of Nurse-Midwifery* states that reducing the number of these visits to 8 affected neither the mother's health nor the pregnancy outcome.

•Again, numerous studies have failed to demonstrate a relationship between sexual intercourse and the onset of labor—either prematurely or at full term. And some of the studies have looked at some remarkably active sexual lifestyles.

•Breast-feeding burns 600–800 maternal calories each and every day.

Diary

My Eighth Month

Problems_____

_____

Medications_____

_____

Illness_____

_____

Rate of baby movement on a scale of 1–10_____

_____

Special tests_____

_____

Natural childbirth classes_____

_____

What's going on in the world?_____

_____

_____

_____

What's going on in my life?_____

_____

_____

_____

My thoughts and feelings_____

_____

_____

_____

Doctor's appointment_____

_____

_____

Questions to ask_____

Nine

My Ninth Lunar Month

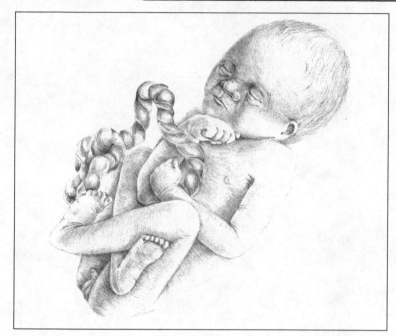

Your baby is within four weeks of full term and weighs around five to six pounds (2,400–2,700 grams). It is about 18 inches (47 centimeters) long. The head is still proportionately larger than the rest of the body and the lower limbs are still shorter than the upper ones. No matter—the great moment is close at hand!

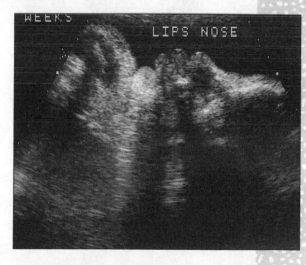

Ultrasound examinations now require many frames to visualize the whole baby, but this is only necessary for special procedures such as a biophysical profile (BPP; see appendix). The frame here shows a profile of a 36-week baby.

Moving right along, you are now in the ninth month of your pregnancy—but you know that better than anyone else. This time frame includes the 32nd to the 36th weeks. A baby born at this time will survive as well as one delivered at term and will be going home with you unless some unexpected complication occurs.

Speaking of home, you probably have made everything ready for your permanent guest, packed and repacked your bag, and had several dry runs to the hospital or birthing center. You have had ten baby showers and received thirty baby outfits, all of which will fit the first week after birth only. All you need now is a little more patience.

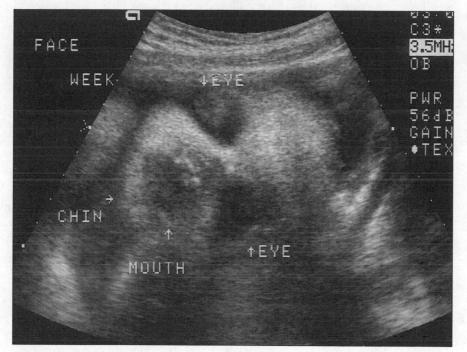

A 36-week fetal face.

Home Births

In recent years, interest in home deliveries has been on the rise, although this interest has apparently not increased the rate of such births, as you will see. Many factors, some of which you know about already, have been responsible for this renewed interest in an old custom. For instance, there is rage and anger in some quarters against a restrictive hospital system that was too slow in responding to the perceived needs of a more liberal and enlightened society. Having all but conquered maternal mortality and made vast inroads in the area of fetal loss, doctors and hospitals were slow to surrender absolute control over the environment and policies that had achieved this remarkable goal. At the same time, similar anger was expressed by a new generation against many societal institutions. This anger reached maximum expression in the 1960s and 1970s, when many dissident citizens did indeed drop out and form their own colonies. Not many of these remain as we enter the next millennium, and certainly, insofar as our institutions are concerned, the hospital environment has vastly changed and is now very responsive to the family unit.

Moreover, having a baby delivered within the system today is expensive, no question about it. Here are the American averages: for the hospital—$1,200 per day; for the obstetrician—$1,570; for the anesthesia—$300; for the pediatrician—$150. These averages are based on a normal delivery and a short hospital stay. Against these figures is the cost of a midwife at home—about $800. Some of us—and some aliens—have no money at all, and certainly not enough for either a delivery at the hospital or a midwife at home. Statistics reveal that depressed areas of our country with a high immigrant population have the highest number of home deliveries. Managed medical care has changed many of these figures, but it has changed nothing for the uninsured.

Back-to-nature movements often made it seem "in" to have a baby at home, and some of your best friends may have done it. The subject usually comes up for discussion at parties just after the football and basketball briefing, but before car-pooling and divorces. The movement now seems to have moved on.

Some very rapid-fire mothers just don't make it in time, and, of course, in certain remote or weather-bound areas of our country it simply takes too long to get to a hospital. As already noted, these are often called "bronco babies"—after the device that tries to get them to a hospital.

The number of out-of-hospital births in the United States has remained more or less constant since 1975. This figure is about 1 percent, and it varies considerably across the United States. In Connecticut and North Dakota, two-tenths of a percent of all deliveries are home births, as compared to Texas with 3 percent, Washington State with 3.5 percent, and Oregon with 4.4 percent.

About one-third of home deliveries are attended by midwives, about one-third by physicians, and one-third by unspecified persons.

As the percentage of hospital births has risen, the rate of infant and maternal death has declined. In 1940, for instance, when 56 percent of all deliveries occurred in hospitals, the infant mortality rate was 47 per 1,000, and the maternal death rate was 376 per 100,000 births. In 1980,

99 percent of all deliveries were in hospitals, the infant mortality rate was 12.4 per 1,000, and the maternal mortality rate 6.9 per 100,000! Today our infant mortality is less than 8 per 1,000 and maternal mortality has remained about the same—an almost irreducible figure that includes many nonobstetrical deaths related to firearms and accidents (see "Prepared Pregnant Pauses" in chapter 8).

It is a myth that home births predominate in other developed countries. In Great Britain, for instance, 98.5 percent of all births occur in hospitals. In Holland—another country often cited for its low infant and maternal mortality rates and high home birth rate—the percentage of hospital deliveries is now over 60 percent and steadily increasing. Those who stay home in Holland are low-risk women who have no other choice, since the government will not pay for their use of hospital facilities.

The belief that childbirth is so safe that it can take place anywhere, and the opposite belief, that all births outside the hospital are unsafe, are probably both untrue. Figures from the National Center on Health Statistics show that 20 percent of women with no underlying medical condition and no previous problem with pregnancy develop some problem during labor. Of these 20 percent, 2 percent represent *acute* problems requiring *immediate* solutions. As an example, shoulder disproportion is not an uncommon delivery event. The head delivers but the shoulders are trapped and require expert management to deliver with safety to both mother and child, a situation that must be resolved quickly—in no more than five minutes. Another example is a prolapsed umbilical cord; this not uncommon event will end tragically within minutes if aggressive treatment is not instituted.

My feelings have probably shown through in this presentation. If you can afford it or are insured, I believe you should go to a family-oriented hospital or birthing center to have your baby.

Gravida . . . Para . . .

You will hear of or read about doctors categorizing pregnant women as *gravid* something, *para* something. It may sound confusing, but it's very simple. *Gravid* or *gravida* refers to the total number of pregnancies a woman has sustained. It doesn't matter whether they were full-term, premature, miscarried, or ectopic—each pregnancy raises gravida by one. *Para, parity,* or *parous* refers to the number of viable deliveries that the gravida has sustained. Thus, a woman who is "gravida four para two" (G4, P2,) has been pregnant four times, with two viable deliveries. This is of little use to you perhaps, but it has some value to us doctors. We use the abbreviations in writing case reports, communicating with other physicians, and keeping hospital records.

Late Examinations by Your Doctor

During the last weeks of your pregnancy, your doctor may examine you internally and may do so more than once. At this time, the size of your pelvis is reevaluated so as to confirm whether its capacity is sufficient to allow passage of your baby's head. One of the reasons this is repeated in late pregnancy is that the baby's head, which is normally the largest part to go through your pelvis, is usually now presenting within the pelvis or close to it. The examination assists in many ways to help evaluate whether your internal measurements are adequate to accept it. The opportunity is also present at this time to determine whether the head is in normal position and coming down well and deep into your pelvis. Finally, such an examination provides an opportunity to evaluate how close to labor you may be. Often the doctor can tell by the condition of your cervix whether labor is imminent or a long way off. Generally, prior to the onset of labor the cervix begins to thin and to open and soften. Sometimes, however, labor begins when the cervix is most unfavorable and unripe.

These late examinations are quite a common and accepted procedure in modern obstetrics. You may spot for many hours afterward, but this should cause no alarm. Very rarely, you may actually bleed, and if this persists or is increasing over a period of several hours, you had better check back.

Admission to Your Birthing Center

Hospitals shouldn't frighten you, particularly modern obstetrical units or birthing centers, and certainly not those that are family-centered and allow free visitation during and after labor. As you already know, the day of closed, off-limits delivery suites and uncaring labor attendants has long since passed. Perhaps you have already toured your own unit during your preparation classes and so are completely familiar with it. If such is the case—and it usually is today—your greatest fear is that you maybe came in too early!

What to Bring

- a small case containing your nightgown, robe, and slippers
- your personal toilet articles—comb, brush, toothbrush, makeup
- a nursing bra and bed jacket
- an outfit for your baby to wear home (a diaper is not necessary)
- the baby's father!

Even if you are staying only one day, bring these items—particularly the last one. If you are not nursing, the hospital usually gives you a 24-hour formula supply to take home with you.

What Not to Bring

Do not bring any personal linens, bath towels, face cloths, sanitary pads, routine baby clothing, or a bunch of relatives. Do not bring much money, and do not bring or wear valuables. Give any jewelry to someone to take home. Remove makeup. If you wear contacts, leave them at home. Spit out your gum!

Some Questions You May Have to Field on Arrival

Most hospitals and birthing centers maintain complete files on expectant mothers who are due to deliver with them. These files are supplied by the doctors and kept in the labor suite so that they will be immediately available should you come in unexpectedly or if for some reason your doctor is not immediately available. Here are the questions:

- your name (don't laugh: You may forget it, or you may give your maiden name—it's happened!)
- your expected date of delivery (EDD)
- your blood type and Rh factor
- pregnancy rank (first, second, and so on)
- your doctor's name
- your pediatrician's name
- whether your membranes have ruptured, and if so, when
- contractions—how often, how long, and where you feel them
- bleeding—amount and color
- baby movement
- last food—what and when
- disposition of contact lenses
- whether you have false teeth or bridges (these may not need to come out, but a delivery table is no place for us to find out that they are there)
- whether you plan to nurse

- any known allergies—to medicine or other substances

- whether X-rays were taken or ultrasound used during pregnancy, and why

- any medical complications or any other information your doctor has advised you to give

Remember the constant plea: If you think you are in labor, *eat nothing*. Drink fluids sparingly or not at all if you are laboring actively.

What Happens in the Hospital or Birthing Center

It is difficult to tell you exactly what will happen here, since there are now so many different techniques of managing labor that all sorts of variables can occur. If you have been privileged to attend classes, however, you already know more or less what will happen at your birthing center. What follows is the basic procedure you are likely to encounter.

First you are examined by a qualified physician or nurse to determine whether you are in labor and to assess your general condition. This examination includes the basics—temperature, pulse, respiratory rate, blood pressure, along with observation of contractions, fetal heart rate and regularity, and evidence of bleeding or ruptured membranes. If it is confirmed that you are in labor or potentially so, or if it is determined that your membranes have truly ruptured, then you are advised to stay. You may have a mini-shave around the vagina, although you can do this yourself at home if your classes have suggested it. Sometimes shaving is omitted. The indignity of a small enema may also be thrust upon you—depending upon a number of circumstances and upon your physician's orders.

After these opening ceremonies, you may go to your birthing room for observation, you may go visit your family, or they may come to you. As labor becomes active, you may be monitored, sedated, have an epidural anesthetic—any of these things may happen depending on the circumstances, the hospital, and the plans you have made with your doctor. Sooner or later you will most likely be connected to intravenous (IV) solutions, which run constantly for the remainder of your labor, delivery, and recovery period. Why these fluids? Here are some good reasons:

- Since your oral fluid intake has terminated and you are working hard (that's why it is called labor), you begin to lose fluid and become dehydrated. This is particularly true in Lamaze labors, which tend to last longer and involve tremendous fluid loss through the lungs (during deep breathing). Intravenous fluids replace the losses in all these cases.

•You also consume energy while you labor, and the sugar in your IV
 fluids conserves your own sugar reserves so that you don't end up
 burning fat. Fat is a poor fuel that produces acidosis while burning.
 Acidosis affects your performance in labor, but also, and most
 importantly, it can produce acidosis in your baby, depressing its
 respiratory centers. The use of sugar in the IV solution, however,
 must be carefully restricted to your immediate needs.

•Medications needed for control of labor, pain, blood pressure, or
 any emergency can be administered through the IV and take effect
 at once. Such medication dosages can be meticulously controlled,
 and thus overdosage and delayed effects can be prevented.

There are other important reasons for giving intravenous fluids during labor, but these are the basic ones. Modern plastic needles are almost
painless, can stay in place for unlimited time, and allow you to move
your arms at will with no significant discomfort.

Sooner or later, either your bed will be converted to a delivery table
or you will go to a delivery room. Then, awake or asleep, your legs are
put into stirrups and, with as much dignity as possible, your bottom is
washed with sterile fluids and covered with drapes. Soon you and your
baby will be separated by a cut in the umbilical cord and then reunited as
he or she is brought to your arms. If your husband, partner, or friend is
with you, fine. If not, and you are awake, you may take your newborn
with you. If for some reason you are asleep or very sedated, someone—
family or attendants—will keep you posted until you can be together. In
most situations, you may hold and cuddle your baby immediately after
birth, and again once he or she has been cleaned and warmed. Your baby
will be left with you and your partner from that point on so that bonding
may proceed.

Finally, you will be taken to a recovery room for an hour or two.
Here specialized attendants can watch your vital signs during this critical
period, observe the contractions of your uterus, and sometimes massage
your abdomen, assisting the contractions in their work of shrinking the
uterus. They make sure that your bladder, with its newfound freedom,
doesn't overfill, and that you are not bleeding excessively for any reason.
In some centers, you will be returned to a private recovery room where
your family can be with you.

When your attendants are sure that you are resting quite normally—
as most likely you will be—you are taken to your room. Hospital visiting
hours in the maternity section are fairly flexible, although visitors other
than family are sometimes excluded when the baby is in the room—
except, of course, for nursing-in arrangements. Most often, fathers may
sleep in. This is entirely good and proper. Nursery-bound babies are reg-

ularly brought out so that father, mother, and baby may enjoy each other. If the newborn is ill and requires confinement to the nursery, then the parents must visit through the viewing window.

Some Questions and Answers About Labor

What starts labor?
A whole series of events must come into play at about the same time in order for labor to start. In the first place, the uterus cannot, regardless of what you may think, go on growing indefinitely, as there are stretch limits to the uterine wall. That is one reason why multiple pregnancies deliver early. Also, the placenta begins to age very rapidly, as shown by the decrease in its progesterone secretion and its ability to transfer oxygen and remove waste products from the unborn infant. The dramatic drop in progesterone is but one of the major triggering factors in the onset of labor. As discussed earlier, the placenta increasingly markets certain agents that signal a change in the oxytocin/oxytocinase system. Oxytocin, secreted by the anterior pituitary gland, is the substance that makes the uterus contract. It is what we give intravenously to induce or augment labor and to make the uterus contract firmly after delivery. Oxytocin is circulated in the bloodstream all the time, but it is inactivated by an equally circulating oxytocinase. Substances secreted by the aging placenta deactivate the oxytocinase, turning the oxytocin loose to set labor in motion.

Labor can also be triggered by PROM—premature rupture of the membranes. The exciting mechanism here is uncertain. Further, labor can be initiated by placental separation. In this dangerous situation, the escaping intrauterine blood acts as a powerful irritant and often produces tetanic uterine contractions.

What about abnormal positions of the baby during labor?
Most commonly, babies come into labor with their heads presenting. Usually at this critical time, the head is well flexed, the chin is on the chest, and the body is lying face down. Sometimes the head is positioned sideways—or even face up. Labor may turn the head to the preferred face-down position, but sometimes the turn must be made forcibly with forceps. This is a skilled art, and it has been replaced many times these days by a cesarean section. The face-down position is important because, in this position, the head diameters are at their smallest while negotiating the mother's bony pelvis.

Breech (bottom first) presentations induce certain hazards during labor and delivery. Many obstetricians feel that the cesarean section is the method of choice in such circumstances. Certain other very abnormal and rare baby presentations—such as hands, shoulders, or backs—must almost always be handled by cesarean section.

What is meant by an incompetent cervical os?
When the cervix fails to remain closed until full term and simply falls open before that time, the resultant disorder is called an incompetent cervical os. Generally it will slip open at the same time in each and every pregnancy sustained by the mother. The incompetence develops as a result of general cervical weakness, cervical tearing during previous deliveries, or surgery to the cervix. Whatever the cause, the internal band of muscle and fibrous tissue that should hold the cervix closed until the full 40 weeks have gone by fails at some time or another. The cervix simply then falls open and the baby is expelled. This occurs generally without any labor and is purely a mechanical defect. If recognized in time, it can often be corrected by sewing the cervix shut with a nylon or similar suture, much like a purse string. This string may be cut when full term is reached, or a cesarean section may be performed and the suture left in place to protect future pregnancies.

What is CPD?
CPD is the abbreviation for cephalo-pelvic disproportion, a situation that arises during labor when the baby's head, because of its size or position, or the mother's pelvis, because of its architecture, hinders passage of the one through the other. Sometimes this can be predicted before the onset of labor; perhaps the maternal bony architecture is very small or has been deformed by disease or injury. Usually, however, one has to await the onset of labor to know whether the disproportion between the baby's head and the mother's pelvis is such that labor cannot progress.

As soon as CPD is identified and the judgment made that it cannot safely be overcome, then delivery, of course, is by cesarean section. Some women are able to deliver one or two children normally and easily and then suddenly develop such CPD that a section is required in the next pregnancy. Such a situation could arise from two circumstances. First, the previous children may have been small—say, between five and six pounds—and the present one weighs nine or ten pounds. Second, the labor may be such that the child's head is presenting in a very abnormal position and simply cannot negotiate the structure of its mother's pelvic canal.

What about the Leboyer method of delivery?
Dr. Frederick Leboyer believes that delivery into this world is a traumatic experience—and so it may be, since the beginning of time. We seem to be well adapted to this trauma, however, since most of us survive without apparent significant personality damage. According to Leboyer, the whole

world might improve if we could have a less traumatic experience at birth. Therefore, he has orchestrated the birth process into a quiet, orderly procedure in which the child is delivered with as little manipulation as possible, with as little lighting as possible, with no attempts to stimulate the child into crying, and with the suppression of any traumatic activity after birth. The child is laid on its mother's abdomen, stroked gently, and treated compassionately. Shortly afterward, it is lowered into a warm bath and encouraged to smile and react in a positive fashion.

Let me hasten to point out that most deliveries today are not conducted as they are on television and on the movie screen. We do not forcibly extract a baby and then beat its bottom in order to make it cry. This is very bad obstetrics—always has been and always will be. Most newborn children are treated gently, and if there is any degree of shock associated with the delivery or the labor, the child is treated with a gentleness and care that you would not believe. In this regard, I couldn't agree more with what Dr. Leboyer preaches, and I and most other practicing obstetricians treat newborns as gently as we can. We do, however, like to see what we are doing and what is happening to the mother, so we prefer to use sufficient light. We also favor a quiet delivery room so that we can concentrate on our work, but we do like to hear the child cry on occasion after birth, particularly since we know that such crying is expanding the terminal sacs of its lungs in preparation for life in the real world. There is basic truth in most fads, but at some point they leave reality and presuppose things that are not proven or don't exist. That's why they don't last.

What is macrosomia?
When the birth weight of a baby exceeds 4,000 grams—about nine pounds—it is called macrosomic. This heavy, large child can cause difficulties during labor and delivery, particularly shoulder dystocia—difficulty in safely extracting the shoulders once the head has been delivered. Macrosomia is generally associated with post-term pregnancies, obese mothers, many previous pregnancies, male babies, previous macrosomia, maternal birth weight, and diabetes. Even with the help of modern ultrasound procedures, macrosomia is difficult to predict with accuracy, but when suspected, preparations should be made for special shoulder care at delivery or the possibility of a cesarean section.

Bonding

The concept of bonding and its application to obstetrics began at Case Western Reserve University's School of Medicine in Cleveland some 20 years ago and since that time has received a great deal of study and interest among physicians and an equal amount of study and interest in the popular press.

Bonding begins in the uterus, where your unborn begins to recognize your voice and your touch. But it is at birth that the relationship can become intense: Now you can see one another, feel, touch, hold, hear clearly, and speak softly to one another, and so come to bond forever. Although this psychological fusion is deepest between mother and child, all members of the family belong in such a bond. Present-day childbirth techniques and hospital environments make bonding a great deal easier to accomplish. Thus, the newborn is placed where both father and mother can touch, feel, and talk with him or her from the moment of birth. In a normal, healthy situation, this close, warm contact is allowed to continue for several hours.

As with all new things, we have to be careful not to carry it to the extreme. The extreme would be making someone feel guilty about not wanting a prolonged bonding experience at birth or, worse still, guilty because of some abnormality in labor and delivery, or about not being able, or allowed, to bond. Thus, from the original concept of bonding as a highly structured and absolutely necessary process for the psychological health of the child, emphasis has now shifted to recognize human adaptability and the possibility of many other successful routes to attachment and, therefore, bonding.

There are many ways parents can become close to and emotionally involved with their babies, and early contact is just one of them. Thus, though bonding is the *ideal* mechanism, it is not the *only* one. No one should feel hurt, ashamed, or guilty over being unable, for whatever reason, to accomplish this goal at the moment of birth. After all, until 20 years ago none of us was even aware of the concept—except mothers and their babes, who have forever been aware of it and have always done it instinctively. Even though they never knew what to call it!

Late Pregnant Pauses

•The word *obstetric* comes from the Latin word *obstare*, a verb meaning "to protect or stand by."

•In 1990 there were 6,179 women members of the American College of Obstetricians and Gynecologists out of a total membership of 30,120. This represents a tripling of the female membership in the last decade. The president of the college in 1984 was Luella Klein, M.D., the first woman to be elected to that office. In 1998 there are 12,504 women members (out of a total membership of 38,776) and the 1998 president will be Vicki L. Seltzer, M.D., from Long Island Jewish Medical Center in New York.

•When it is known that blood will be needed at a planned cesarean section (for a placenta previa, for instance), mothers may donate their own blood to hold in reserve for the operation. Such blood needs to be drawn no later than two weeks prior to the expected surgery. About one mother in 50 faints (vaso-vagal reaction) at the time of donation, versus one in 100 nonpregnant donors. No unusual fetal effects have been noted to follow such donations. Of course, the mother must not be anemic to begin with!

•The number of hospitals providing maternity care decreased from 4,163 in 1981 to 3,545 in 1992. The closing of smaller facilities was responsible for most of this decrease. In 1992 just 9 percent of all deliveries were carried out in small (less than 500 deliveries per year) units; 27 percent were in medium (500–1,499 deliveries) units; and the remaining 64 percent took place in large units (over 1,500 deliveries per year). The larger units had much more specialized maternal and infant care and in-house rather than on-call anesthesia services. During these study years, the use of general anesthesia declined greatly and that of epidurals doubled.

•If your baby is driving you up a wall, you need some adult conversation with others in the same soup, and you are on the Internet, try: http://www.parent soup.com

Diary

My Ninth Month

Problems_____

Medications_____

_____

_____

Rate of baby's movement on a scale of 1–10_____

_____

_____

Special tests_____

_____

_____

Natural childbirth classes_____

_____

What's going on in the world?_____

_____

_____

_____

What's going on in my life?_____

_____

_____

_____

My thoughts and feelings_____

_____

_____

_____

Doctor's appointment_____

_____

_____

Questions to ask_____

_____

_____

_____

_____

_____

_____

_____

_____

_____

_____

_____

_____

_____

_____

_____

_____

_____

_____

_____

_____

_____

_____

_____

_____

_____

_____

Ten

My Tenth Lunar Month

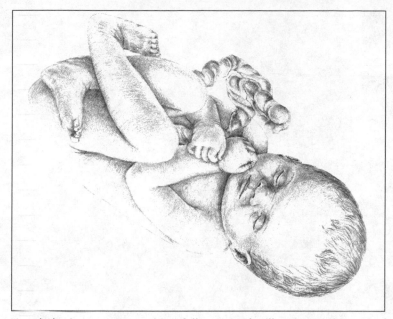

Your baby is now approaching full term and will arrive at the end of this month—give or take a week or two! The average weight of a term newborn is seven pounds (3,150 grams) and it measures close to 20 inches (52 centimeters) in overall length. There are, however, wide variations in these normal measurements. Lanugo hair is completely gone and nails are about ready for trimming. Every important body system is ready to go—and that includes its lungs and vocal cords!

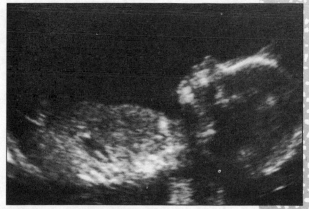

Taken on a high-resolution machine, this very unusual full-term ultrasound was able to capture a great deal more of the baby's body than expected. The ultrasound on page 241 displays the usual amount of head and neck profile visible at 40 weeks.

This is it! You are about to enter the tenth and last lunar month of your pregnancy—the 36th to the 40th weeks. Hallelujah! By now you have read this book until you are sick of it, your nursery is ready, your prenatal classes are finished, your hospital route has been identified, your instructions for labor are clear, your mate is on red-alert, and all else is in readiness. Or is it? Things are usually so complex at this time that you may not know whether to go to the bathroom, put the door back on the microwave, or wind your watch!

If you have had any unusual vaginal infections, your obstetrician may take some special tests early this month. You will be visiting her or his office weekly by now, and there should be an opportunity to talk over any worries you have about the upcoming event or to report any unusual symptoms. You should be continuing to observe your baby's movements. It ought to be kicking about ten times each hour, and you may want to set aside one hour each day to count them. It is very important to tell your doctor if you feel the kick count is declining.

Although the average infant birth weight at full term is about seven pounds, there is a great deal of individual variation: The usual range is from five and a half to nine pounds. Anything below that is called premature—although, as you already know, it may not be—and anything above that is

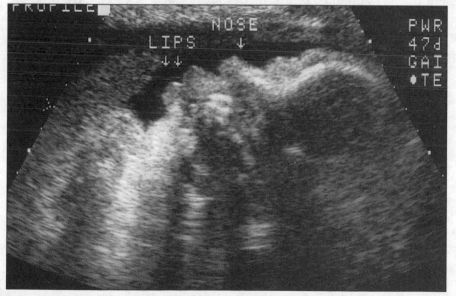

A fetal face in profile at 40 weeks.

considered macrosomic—and you already know that, too. So what? You're still wearing the same old rags and still have a love/hate relationship with the bathroom. Incidentally, the largest newborn baby recorded in all reasonably documented history weighed 26 pounds net, but be consoled: It is truly exceptional for a baby to weigh over 13 pounds at birth. Again, you already know that the birth weight of a newborn child is a function of a combination of factors—its genetic or inherited background, the total duration of the pregnancy, the diet that carried you through pregnancy, and certain complicating factors, such as diabetes, which may greatly affect the size of the baby. Remember, although you are technically due at the end of this month, in a normal pregnancy you are not overdue for two more weeks beyond that point. I didn't write the rules.

Anesthesia and Analgesia

In 1992 the American College of Obstetricians and Gynecologists, in conjunction with the American Society of Anesthesiologists, issued a statement on pain during labor, which includes the following: "Labor results in severe pain for many women. There is no other circumstance where it is considered acceptable for a person to experience severe pain amenable to safe intervention, while under a physician's care." It is notable that both sexes are well represented in each of these organizations (see "Late Pregnant Pauses," chapter 9).

Interestingly, most of the research done about pain relief during labor and delivery and most of the applications of that research have been the product of men's labor. We've already talked about that just a bit. Also, it was a man who first insisted that women be allowed pain relief during labor and who first introduced it to the birthing rooms—although Queen Victoria, as we learned earlier, gave ether a mighty imperial boost when she insisted on having it at her disposal while delivering her son Edward— known in later life as Edward the Peacemaker, the great British monarch whose wit and wisdom seemed blunted not at all by his mother's acceptance of this powerful pain-relieving agent while delivering him!

At any rate, no male physician in history, including this one, ever has had or ever will have the fortune or misfortune to experience childbearing and its pain—or lack of it. Also, we didn't introduce pain relief against our patients' will or to take advantage of them in whatever way while they were in a drug-induced trance. The early church and many laypeople said that we did—but we didn't. We did it for our patients. Now, of course, pain relief is an integral part of labor and delivery and a most important aspect of modern obstetrics. It is more than a matter of providing comfort to the mother; it is an absolute and necessary part of good obstetrical practice. Thoughtfully chosen analgesia can improve labor, and proper anesthesia permits difficult deliveries to be accomplished with safety and comfort.

Before proceeding further, we need to define some terms.

- **Analgesia** is actually stage 1 of general anesthesia. At this point, memory is suspended and the patient experiences varying degrees of insensitivity to pain or lack of perception of pain. Yet she is sufficiently conscious to allow protective reflexes to function—for instance, she can still swallow and close her vocal cords.

- **Anesthesia** is full loss of sensation. General anesthesia involves not only loss of sensation but loss of consciousness, motor power, and reflex activity. Local or regional anesthesia produces loss of pain sensation and motor activity by blocking sensory impulses in a given region of the body. There are many forms of regional anesthesia. In obstetrics they include large or major blocks, such as a spinal or epidural block, both of which are given in the lower back and are very effective; and lesser blocks, such as local infiltrations in the perineum and into the cervical area. Either general or regional anesthesia can provide suitable conditions for most normal and operative obstetrical procedures.

Now then, as the opening paragraph of this section states, and as anyone who has ever been on either end of the delivery table, and who is not a fanatic, would agree, some parts of labor and delivery are very painful. We've been over that, too. There are several variables that determine the amount of pain felt:

- **Individual pain threshold.** It takes more pain to make some of us *feel* it.

- **Fear.** A painful experience that is feared is doubly, triply, or exponentially more painful. Therefore, healthy preparation for childbirth helps dispel fear and so reduce pain. This is one of the great contributions of prepared childbirth classes. Every expectant mother would immensely profit by attending such a class, at least during her first pregnancy.

- **Abnormal labor.** When an abnormal presentation occurs—a breech or a badly extended head or a tight fit—labor may be long, arduous, and filled with pain. Such a labor without pain relief is unconscionable in our society.

As mentioned, childbirth education, provided properly, results in less need for pharmacological pain relief. However, you should *not* be made to feel guilty or ashamed if you choose to utilize an acceptable mode of pharmacological pain relief as labor progresses. This has been mentioned earlier in our discussions on prepared childbirth but deserves mention again. If someone makes you feel that way, back off—you are dealing with a fanatic and a nut.

Obstetrical Pain Relief Principles

Significant discomfort in the early stages of labor is usually managed by the use of a variety of drugs. Most generally these drugs include narcotics and tranquilizers, provided in doses that are considered safe for the infant. In past years, these agents were used together in large doses to produce what was known as "twilight sleep." The dosages at that time were quite a bit greater than they are today, and the use of these drug combinations fell into disfavor when more and more women wished or agreed to participate actively in their labor and delivery. The use of these agents, however, was characterized by a rather wide safety margin for both the mother and the fetus and generally were well handled by both. Today some or all of these agents are still used in the very early stages of labor—again, in more modest doses—and then followed, if possible, by a regional anesthetic, either an epidural or a spinal. If deeper anesthesia is needed and for some reason regional anesthesia cannot be given, then a balanced inhalation anesthetic must be used.

General Anesthesia

Balanced general anesthesia consists of the use of intravenous barbiturates to induce the anesthesia, accompanied by inhalation of nitrous oxide and oxygen to maintain unconsciousness.

The addition of intravenous succinylcholine—a muscle paralyzer—produces deep enough anesthesia and relaxation so that even a very difficult cesarean section can be performed quite readily, and certainly any operative vaginal procedure can also be accomplished. The advantage of general versus conduction anesthesia is that it can be given by nurse anesthetists, who in many obstetrical units are more readily available than physician anesthesiologists.

Besides the general availability of inhalation anesthesia, another advantage is that it displays a wide margin of safety in terms of transfer of the anesthetic agents across the placenta and, therefore, respiratory depression of the newborn infant. But there is no question that anesthetic agents do have a certain amount of depressant effect upon the newborn, particularly if the anesthesia has gone on for a long time.

Finally, inhalation anesthesia tends to induce vomiting. This is not a problem for patients who are well prepared for anesthesia, but many laboring mothers are not well prepared and have food in the stomach when they come to deliver. This is one of the reasons we caution you not to eat if you even *think* you are in labor. Even if you haven't eaten recently, gastric emptying time is delayed in early labor, and thus food tends to stay in the stomach for many hours after it has been eaten.

General anesthesia is being used less and less frequently in obstetrical units as regional anesthesia improves and becomes more readily available. It is generally used only when nothing else is available or great haste is required.

Regional Anesthesia

There are five categories of regional anesthesia:

1. **Spinal block.** This procedure involves placing a needle within the membranes (dura) that surround the spinal nerve cord, extracting a small amount of the enclosed spinal fluid, and replacing it with anesthesia agents. The patient experiences almost instantaneous numbness and motor paralysis from that point in the spinal canal downward. Sometimes the same reaction extends higher into the spinal canal, depending upon the type of agent used. The advantage of a spinal block is that it produces instantaneous pain relief virtually all the time, and it has no effect upon the fetus whatsoever—provided that the mother's blood pressure is kept within acceptable levels at all times. There is a tendency for blood pressure to fall when any major block anesthetic procedure is instituted. The disadvantage of a spinal anesthetic is that the effective duration is short—usually the maximum is two hours. Until very recently, a headache lasting for several days or even weeks followed about 2 percent of all patients treated with spinal anesthesia. The headaches are due to a tiny leak in the membranes (dura) surrounding the spinal cord—a leak from the spot where the spinal needle pierces the dura. There are ways of patching these dural leaks so as to arrest post-spinal headaches, but they are not always successful and the headache may have to run its course of several days. The recent introduction of very small spinal needles, however, has eliminated most headaches completely.

2. **Epidural block or lumbar epidural block.** Another form of regional anesthesia that produces pain relief and some degree of motor loss, this anesthetic is given in a small area just outside the dura in the epidural space. Usually a tiny catheter is inserted into this area, and the anesthetic is administered and readministered through it for as long as necessary to complete labor and delivery. One of its advantages, therefore, is that it can be given relatively early in labor

and continued throughout the remainder of labor and delivery. Another real advantage is that it's not followed by a headache. It is generally safe and well tolerated by a laboring mother, and it allows her to participate to a distinct degree in the birthing process and to watch her delivery and bond with her baby afterward. The disadvantages of lumbar blocks are few. One major problem is that an anesthesiologist or obstetrician must administer it. Although in many obstetrical units the nurse anesthetist can follow the progress of a block once it has been administered by a physician, it still must be placed by a physician.

Very seldom are there any fetal effects from an epidural anesthetic. One temporary problem is a reaction to the anesthetic agent used. Some of the medication always gets into the maternal circulation, and therefore the fetal circulation, where it is known to concentrate. This can affect the infant's heart rate; if it does, delivery is postponed until the effect wears off. This event, incidentally, can be followed quite easily in a monitored labor. Also, as with spinal anesthetics, there is a tendency for hypotension or low blood pressure to follow epidural anesthetic administration. This must be carefully watched for and treated properly by correct positioning of the laboring mother and adjustment of her fluid and medicine intake to keep her blood pressure stable.

Occasionally epidural anesthesia retards labor, and so it must be augmented with pitocin. On the other hand, epidural anesthesia sometimes accelerates the progress of labor. Epidural anesthesia has been repeatedly accused of increasing the section rate by interfering with normal labor progress. There is no substantial evidence that such is the case. Epidurals given for a section can be continued for at least 24 hours after delivery and pain control can be delivered through this source without maternal sedation. All in all, this particular form of regional anesthesia is probably the most popular type of obstetrical anesthetic pain relief in use today.

3. **Combined spinal-epidural block.** This is a very new procedure with many supporters. It involves the administration of a narcotic drug through the new tiny spinal needle, followed later by an epidural using a combination of agents that prevent pain but still allow mobility. Both insertions are made through just one anesthetized skin spot. This technique provides rapid onset of pain relief while allowing the laboring mother to walk about during labor, thus giving her a greater sense of control. The major question remains: Does this procedure, like straight epidurals, increase the cesarean section rate? Again, there is no *substantial* answer yet.

4. **Pudendal block.** This is a local block given into the perineum and the areas that surround the vagina and cervix. It is administered by the obstetrician just prior to delivery and gives adequate local anesthesia for the use of outlet forceps and performance of an episiotomy. It is of no value in any form of operative intervention. It has practically no effect on the infant unless large amounts of the local agent somehow get into the maternal circulation.

5. **Paracervical block.** This technique is also very local. As the name indicates, local anesthesia agents are injected on either side of the cervix to produce, again, local blocks of pain conduction. Its disadvantages are almost identical to those of the pudendal variety, although it is more likely to produce temporary depression of the fetal heart rate, since more of it is likely to get into the maternal circulation.

These, then, are the common agents used in obstetrics to produce analgesia and anesthesia during labor and delivery. You can see that each has its pros and cons, and that there is a place for any of them under the right circumstances. Long before you go into labor you will more than likely have discussed your pain relief options with your doctor. He or she will ask you what type of pain relief you wish, if any, and will bring up any peculiarities of your particular pregnancy that might make the choice of one over another form of anesthesia more rational. Undoubtedly, this subject will come up several times during the course of your prenatal visits.

Anesthesia for Cesarean Section

Either regional or general anesthesia may be used for a cesarean section delivery. Many times an epidural anesthetic is in place and functioning when the decision is made to do a cesarean section, and so it may simply be continued. However, there are times when regional anesthesia is not the choice and a general anesthetic is required. A regional anesthetic would be favored if the patient to be sectioned has a full stomach, a respiratory infection or respiratory disease, or some other anticipated airway difficulty. On the other hand, a general anesthetic is preferred if a rapid delivery is indicated—such as when the uterus is in a constant contraction for whatever reason, or there is excessive maternal bleeding, a clotting disorder, a prolapsed umbilical cord, or certain maternal neurological disorders. All these and more justify general anesthesia for delivery.

So, in operative obstetrics there is room—and, indeed, a need—for both general and regional anesthetic procedures. Again, your doctor will

surely discuss the advantages and disadvantages of any particular anesthetic with you and will use, with your consent, the one most suitable to
your needs.

Labor — Downloading

Labor is the forceful expulsion of a baby and its placenta from the uterus
through the vagina. It normally begins within a week or two on either
side of day 265. In the first pregnancy it usually lasts about 12 hours,
and in subsequent pregnancies 6 to 8 hours. There are wide variations,
however, within all these limits. We will talk about prolonged labor
shortly. True labor begins when the cervix begins active dilation and not
necessarily with the onset of regular cramps.

False Labor

During the last few weeks of pregnancy, the uterus is contracting with
considerable vigor, and it is not unusual for some of the contractions to
be moderately painful. If, as occasionally happens, these episodes become
regular and really uncomfortable, you might be dealing with false labor.
The contraction pattern in false labor may be very regular, that is, you
may have contractions at five-minute intervals, lasting about half a
minute, and this may go on for many hours. But there are several differences between false and true labor—differences not always easy to assess.

- •False labor goes nowhere. No matter how long it continues, there is
  no dilation of the cervix. Only true labor accomplishes this.
  Clearly, this is a difference you cannot determine.

- •Although the contractions may be regular and uncomfortable,
  generally the interval between them remains about the same no matter
  how long the pains last. Thus, if at the end of four hours the interval
  is still five minutes, you are most likely experiencing false labor.

- •The contractions of false labor eventually disappear or can be made
  to disappear with mild sedatives or pain medication.

- •With false labor, there is no bloody discharge and no rupture of the
  membranes. Either of those signs indicates labor.

Despite these clues, it is often difficult to tell false from true labor,
and you most certainly must consult your doctor if you are in doubt.
Even he or she may not be sure and may ask you to come to the office or
the hospital to be checked carefully in order to determine exactly what is
going on.

True Labor

True labor usually begins with the same sort of menstrual-like cramps that herald the onset of a period, often beginning in your lower back and swinging around into your lower abdomen. Frequently such cramps are as much as half an hour apart, but they soon get closer, longer, and harder. Your doctor will probably want you to call when the contractions are about eight to ten minutes apart—unless your membranes rupture before that time or unless there is some obstetrical reason you have been asked to call earlier.

In rare instances, labor begins suddenly, with contractions that are very close together and produce real discomfort. Under these circumstances, you should call and then prepare to take off pronto. Finally, labor may begin with or be preceded by a discharge of bloody mucus, called show. You need not call your doctor if show appears, since active labor may be hours away, but if you have any heavy bleeding from the vagina, call immediately.

Occasionally the membranes rupture before labor begins or during early labor. Fluid gushes from the vagina or trickles constantly and uncontrollably. When you feel that your membranes have ruptured, you should report it to your doctor and put down the pizza. Very, very rarely, a tragic accident may happen when the membranes rupture. If the baby is not sitting well in the pelvis or is in an abnormal position, the umbilical cord may prolapse when the membranes rupture. Should that occur—and again, it is exceedingly rare—enough umbilical cord may come down that you can feel or see it protruding from your vagina. In that event, feel to be sure that it is pulsating—as long as it is pulsating, your baby will be fine. Even if you cannot be sure about pulsations, you must lie down immediately and put several pillows under your bottom to keep the baby's presenting part from dropping into the pelvis. Your head, upper body, and abdomen should be considerably below your pelvis and lower extremities. Someone else must call an ambulance and get you to a hospital in that same position, maintaining constant vigilance to be sure that the cord is continuing to pulsate. Again, this is a most unusual happenstance, but quick treatment can prevent a catastrophe. And even if the cord has not come down far enough to be seen, sudden violent baby activity within your uterus after the membranes rupture might indicate that this rare event has taken place. Again, prop your bottom half up and get help.

The Stages of Labor

The expulsion of your child into the world by labor is divided into three stages. The cascade of labor is, first, to force open (dilate) the cervix completely; to push the presenting part, usually the head, through the maternal pelvis; and to deliver the baby out to the world—probably the shortest and most hazardous trip your child will ever take!

In the **first** stage of labor, the cervix dilates completely. Labor usually begins with the cervix somewhere between one and three centimeters (between a half-inch and an inch) dilated. Complete dilation—ten centimeters—usually requires some eight to ten hours in the first pregnancy, often considerably less in subsequent pregnancies. During this time, the presenting part, usually the head, is most likely descending into and through the pelvic canal. Dilation of the cervix is accomplished in effect by reduction of the volume in the uterine cavity. The uterine contractions you felt throughout most of your pregnancy might be likened to flexing your arm—tightening the muscles, then letting the arm straighten and relaxing the whole muscle. Now that labor has begun, the contractions change in a very significant way. Each time the muscles tighten, they grow a little shorter. Comparing it to your arm again, each time you flex the muscle, your elbow bends a little more, until finally your hand is touching your shoulder. Thus, in the uterine cavity, as the muscle fibers grow shorter, the capacity of the uterus to contain your baby diminishes and so it pushes against the cervix to find a way out. The cervix, being properly prepared, dilates to provide that way out.

During the first stage of labor, there is no advantage to voluntary pushing or bearing down, nor should you feel any desire to do so. Such muscular activity would only exhaust you, and you cannot push a baby through an unopened cervix any more than you can push yourself through an unopened door. You are generally receiving fluids intravenously at this time. Most likely a monitor is attached to your abdomen. You may have been given some medication for pain relief, depending upon your wishes, your preparedness, and your perceived pain. If you are going to have an epidural anesthetic, it is customarily administered when dilation has reached three to four centimeters (two inches), but this may be delayed if your labor is very slow, the baby is not descending well into your pelvis, or you have no particular desire for pain relief at this time. If you are following a prepared childbirth program, you are directing all your efforts during the first stage of labor toward achieving the utmost in relaxation and the conversion of pain sensation to other sensations.

In the *second* stage of labor, the cervix is completely dilated and the baby needs to be pushed out into the world. This may take a minute, or it may take several hours. Generally, the more babies you have had, the quicker it takes place. If you have received no anesthesia, you will experience an intense urge to bear down, such as you would during a bowel movement. It is at this time that the voluntary muscular system comes into play, and actively pushing and bearing down with your abdominal muscles can be of great assistance.

If you have had an epidural anesthetic, you will have no feeling what-soever at this time. The contractions of the uterus as it continually decreases in size continue to force the baby through the pelvic canal and out into your doctor's waiting hands. In order to shorten the second stage, particularly if there is an abnormal presentation of the head, it may be necessary to use forceps to turn the head or simply to ease it over the entrance of the vagina. Regardless of what you may have heard, for-ceps applications are very safe in skilled hands. Your doctor may also perform an episiotomy (see page 254) during the final phase of the sec-ond stage. Your baby, if he or she is well, will be given to you so that bonding may begin.

The *third* stage of labor consists of placental expulsion. This can hap-pen very abruptly after delivery of the child, or it may require many min-utes and some assistance. A number of doctors are now removing the placenta manually after the delivery, but many still wait for the natural separation to occur and for the placenta to slip out by itself. There is nothing one can do to aid in this stage of labor. You are probably not even thinking about it as you cuddle your newborn child. Very frequently before the placenta delivers, routine samples of blood are taken from the umbilical cord to be sent to the laboratory to determine the baby's blood type and whether any significant antibodies are present, as well as to do other blood tests if indicated. For instance, if the baby was depressed for any reason at birth, the doctor would probably want to get blood oxygen and carbon dioxide saturation as well as a ph determination in order to evaluate the degree of depression or acidosis. Also, as we shall see, cord blood is now being collected and stored by some families as a source of future stem cells to avoid bone marrow transplants in certain cases of cancer—both in the newborn and in other family members.

But to move on—sooner or later the placenta is delivered and your labor is finished. Your doctor then explores the birth canal for any retained tissue or membranes and evidence of any birth canal tear. If all is well, he or she repairs your episiotomy—if you sustained one—and you are on your own again. Your true labor, however, is just beginning—it is gurgling now upon your chest.

Soon the adorable little creature will be separated from you for a few minutes. He or she will have two Apgar scores (see the glossary and "Pregnant Pauses" at the end of this chapter) recorded—the first at one minute and the second at five minutes. Your baby will also be cleaned up a bit and wrapped in swaddling clothes before being returned to your arms for you and your partner to admire; if he is not with you in the delivery room, you are then wheeled out to show your baby to him and to the world.

In the unlikely event that your baby is not quite stable at birth, he or she will be whisked off—once you have seen and touched him or her—to a neonatal intensive-care unit for very special care until stability is attained.

Again, this warning: If you think you are in labor, or if your membranes have ruptured, *do not eat or drink* anything from that moment on. Call your doctor for further instructions.

Prolonged Labor

This is a very difficult topic to talk about and to quantify. In the past, certain exact time constraints were put on the total length of labor before it became prolonged—such as 18 hours in the first labor and 12 hours in all subsequent labors. For a number of reasons, such limits don't work out. Earlier we saw that the first labor usually lasts some 12 hours or more and subsequent ones between six and eight hours—all of these being estimated figures. There may be significant variation both up and down with these figures and yet all remains normal, depending upon many circumstances.

What we look for is a labor that is progressing regularly and picking up steam as middle to late first-stage labor is approached. The so-called Friedman curve demonstrates the progress of normal labor over any time frame. Interruptions or arrests along that curve are what give us concern in any labor. Thus, we are more concerned with arrests than with actual time—although both are significant.

Prolonged labor has several causes:

- **Uterine inertia.** When uterine labor contractions are inefficient or irregular, then progress is slow. Such inertia—the inability to get moving—may be caused by oversedation, twins or more, many previous pregnancies, or fear. Contraction stimulation with pitocin usually resolves the problem before labor becomes very prolonged.

- **Arrest.** This is really the worrisome problem—a labor that began very properly but at some point arrested. Most often arrest is due to a problem between the baby's head and the mother's pelvis (see CPD, page 233). The situation may correct itself spontaneously as the baby molds a bit to conform to the passageway. Nevertheless, a great deal of judgment and close observation are necessary because sometimes that adjustment will not safely take place. Rather than have a prolonged labor, which is not good for either participant, a cesarean section is in order.

The Induction of Labor

To induce labor is to purposely set in motion the process of labor at a selected time preceding the onset of natural labor. There are two types of induced labor: indicated and elective.

•An **indicated** induction is undertaken when some condition of the mother or her unborn child (or both) makes early delivery necessary. Severe hypertension of pregnancy or a positive contraction stress test (see the appendix) are typical reasons for an indicated induction. Such an induction must sometimes be attempted as much as a month before the baby is due, and because there is no time to prepare for the normal labor cascade, it is often difficult and dangerous. However, the risks of waiting longer are even greater. Indicated inductions used to be called forced labor.

•An **elective** induction presupposes that the pregnancy is perfectly normal, that the mother is at full term and her baby is a good size, and that all conditions are favorable for a regular delivery. This, then, is a convenience type of delivery. An elective induction makes it easier for the mother to make her arrangements at home, get to the hospital in comfort—especially if she labors rapidly—and be certain that the hospital and delivery room crew are at full strength. Since these deliveries are for the convenience of the mother, her family, and the doctor, it is extremely important that no greater risk be incurred than if the labor were to occur naturally.

In well-documented studies of thousands upon thousands of controlled elective inductions of labor, it has been shown beyond doubt that the intelligent induction of labor by a skilled practitioner carries with it less risk to both mother and child than does spontaneous labor. It should be emphasized, however, that the mother must be selected carefully for this procedure and the doctor must be skilled in the induction of labor.

Some elective inductions are almost indicated. Consider a mother who lives a remote distance from her hospital, may not always have ready transportation, may have weather problems, and may labor rapidly. Almost any of these conditions would merit an elective procedure. And one final benefit—mother arrives prepared, with dignity, and hungry!

Elective inductions are being performed somewhat less often in this country because of quality assurance programs and the charged medicolegal climate. Anything that goes wrong, regardless of its relevance, may become the burden of the inducer.

In the usual course of events in an induction, you go to the hospital in the early morning hours with an empty stomach. An intravenous catheter is set in place and fluids started. Pitocin—the great uterine stimulator—is then gradually and carefully metered into the IV and your resultant contractions monitored along with the fetal heart rate. If it is proper, the membranes are ruptured early on. If you are having an epidural, it will be given when you are moving along satisfactorily. And so it goes.

Sometimes when an indicated induction is being done, an unfavorable cervix may be softened and labor enhanced by the vaginal insertion of prostaglandin creams or suppositories. These insertions take place well before the induction is started.

Episiotomy

We have seen that, during the second stage of labor, your child is pushed out into the world. Although the vagina is capable of a great deal of stretching, the muscles and skin that make it up can and do tear and sustain certain damage at the time of delivery. Most often during your first delivery, and perhaps in some of those that follow, your doctor will do an episiotomy, that is, make an incision into the muscles and skin of the vagina, and the skin on the outside as well, in order to prevent a tear. After your child and the placenta are delivered, this incision is a clean, straight wound that is easy to repair, whereas a tear would be jagged and rough and difficult to repair decently. Occasionally an episiotomy is not necessary because tissues stretch satisfactorily or have already been stretched by a previous delivery.

Although your episiotomy may cause you some discomfort after you deliver, it heals much better than a tear and gives you much better support for later years. Most episiotomies are repaired with suture material that dissolves and does not have to be removed after delivery. One of the most common questions a doctor is asked after delivery is: "How many stitches were used to repair my episiotomy?" This is a difficult question to answer, for many of our suture techniques resemble hemstitching, that is, we use one continuous suture throughout most or all of the episiotomy, taking small stitches just as you would in hemming a skirt. This works much better than basting the incision or taking a couple of big stitches. (A suture, then, may consist of a single separate stitch or a number of running stitches.) Therefore, the answer to that question is meaningless. Believe me, it is better to have 100 small stitches than two great big grabbers.

Lately the episiotomy, like so many other elements of pregnancy and childbirth, has fallen victim to the frantic race among some of the cultists to get motherhood back to nature before things get too good. Many women who do not receive an intervention like a proper episiotomy tend to develop several specific disorders from the resultant muscle and skin damage that will require intervention sometime in the future. Relaxation of the vagina can also lead to a loss of sexual sensation. This loss of sexual sensation is felt (or not felt) by both partners. Although the back-to-nature movement is a well-intended, highly motivated effort to attain, through education and training, certain psychological goals, the goal of anti-episiotomy adherents remains obscure.

Forceps

Although I said that forceps were introduced by a doctor in the last century and incidentally revolutionized obstetrics, that statement is probably not entirely correct. It is altogether likely that forceps of a sort were invented in ancient times but that the techniques were lost for centuries thereafter.

Modern forceps are still used to extract babies mechanically from their mothers. Forceps deliveries are the so-called instrument deliveries. When they were first used, forceps were reserved for the most difficult obstructed labors, and the results, as might be imagined, were not too good. Today forceps are used primarily to shorten the second stage of labor and reduce the prolonged pounding of the baby's head against the mother's tissues. The use of forceps in this situation is not dangerous, and it harms neither the mother nor the child in any known way.

Occasionally forceps have to be used to turn a baby who is lying abnormally in the mother's pelvis, thus causing progress in labor to cease. Such forceps deliveries are considerably more difficult to execute and, as time goes by, are becoming a vanishing art. Cesarean section now often replaces the difficult forceps rotation in cases of arrested position.

Another type of instrument delivery is used in many areas of this country and abroad. It is called a *vacuum extractor* and—pardon the comparison—works something like a plumber's helper! A rubber or plastic cup is applied to the infant's head, and a suction device produces a vacuum between the head and the extractor. The physician then uses this to put gentle traction on the child's head and turn and deliver it through the pelvis. The advocates of this device say that it is less likely to damage the child or the mother's small parts, and they certainly have a good argument. The instrument will probably be used increasingly to assist in the termination of the second stage of labor.

Overdue?

The last time we talked about being overdue, you had just missed a period; now you are missing a baby! Although you have been told that you are not overdue until you have gone at least two weeks beyond the expected date of delivery, as far as you are concerned, you were overdue at midnight yesterday. Your family and in-laws and all your friends feel the same way and very frequently express this conviction. But they are wrong.

In a normal, healthy pregnancy, the onset of labor may occur anywhere from two weeks before to two weeks after the expected day of delivery. And that is a fact.

One of the problems we face in dating a pregnancy is that we are not always certain of the exact duration of the pregnancy, and even the two people involved are not often absolutely certain when the fruitful union took place. The information we must assess to determine the correct dates includes the date when contraception ceased, the date of the last menstrual period, the determination of pregnancy duration on your first pelvic examination, the appearance of an audible heartbeat, and the rate of uterine growth as pregnancy advanced. Two specific tests that may be of great help are the HCG pregnancy test—which, if done very early in pregnancy, is a really good indicator of pregnancy duration—and, of course, an ultrasound, which is probably the greatest help of all. (Turn to the appendix to learn how ultrasound can determine pregnancy duration.)

Should the pregnancy last beyond 42 weeks—proven—it becomes a different problem entirely. Not only is it now called a post-mature or post-date pregnancy, but it is subject to very close observation by the responsible physician. Five percent of all pregnancies end up here, and they are supported by a placenta that reached its maturity around the 37th pregnancy week. As this placenta ages, we are very concerned about its ability to nourish and oxygenate the fetus on the far end of its journey.

Because of the increasing placental senescence, most obstetricians will induce labor at the end of the 42nd week. If the induction conditions are not reasonably favorable at this time, the pregnancy must be watched very closely and tests for fetal well-being routinely performed. Such tests include the nonstress test, the contraction stress test, a biophysical profile, amniocentesis, assessment of blood hormone levels, and so forth (see the appendix). If these show any evidence of fetal stress and the cervix is still unfavorable, the physician will probably decide to deliver by cesarean section, although the new prostaglandin cervical softening agents may work (see The Induction of Labor, pages 252–254). No matter what the circumstances, a pregnancy is not likely to be allowed to persist undelivered for very long after the onset of the third proven post-date week. Your obstetrician may not follow my plan exactly as outlined, but the principles remain the same.

Room and Bored

In those lazy hazy days of the recent past, women luxuriated in the hospital for ten days or so, even after the most uneventful delivery! Clean sheets, twice-daily back rubs, good food and no dishes to wash, baby away somewhere in a distant nursery getting fed, washed, changed, and spoiled by some nurse—it was a piece of cake! Seems foolish for you to have taken up arms against treatment like that, doesn't it?

Well, ten days in the hospital would bankrupt most young families today, and besides, it wasn't all as good as it sounds. Those mothers were kept in bed too long and suffered a multitude of problems because of it, some of them very serious. Anyway, those days are gone forever, and the average postpartum stay is now about one whole day or, in the case of a section, about two whole days. You are usually out of the birthing compound before your bed linens have been changed or the ink is dry on your admission sheet!

What goes on in those few hours? Well, it's not boring anymore—there isn't time. Indeed, if your baby is rooming in, a little boredom would be welcome. Dad is with you part of the time, and your baby all the time. Even if you do not have rooming-in, it is still a pretty busy place. Visitors will be in to see you, depending upon your hospital's regulations. It is good to abide by these regulations, since they are meant to protect you and your baby, and sometimes there can be too many good things and good visitors! Visitors often forget their social etiquette and overstay. Fortunately, none can smoke anymore, since almost every hospital in our country is smoke-free.

Hospital schedules are funny, to say the least; they may seem to be arranged for the convenience of doctors and nurses—and that may be partly true. So you may be getting up when you used to go to bed and eating your evening meal during the soaps! Incidentally, some hospitals give the new parents a champagne dinner the first night after delivery. Even if your hospital does not, they probably wouldn't mind if somebody brought this celebration to you. Like Dad.

Here are some things to observe about your own body functions during the precious-few lying-in hours that are left to you:

- You will have a bloody vaginal discharge no matter how you delivered. This discharge is called lochia. It may be heavier than a period at first but rapidly diminishes over the first few days. Sanitary pads must be worn—you cannot use a tampon until your doctor says you can, which will be a few weeks away. Lochia comes from the uterus, mainly the placental site; as the uterus shrinks to normal size over the next two weeks, the bleeding decreases. It may not stop completely until many weeks have gone by.

- You may have been catheterized to remove urine from your bladder. This may have been done during labor and again at delivery. Because of this and the stresses put on your bladder during labor and delivery, it is not uncommon to have mild discomfort on voiding. Sometimes the bladder is temporarily paralyzed and an indwelling catheter must be inserted and left for a day or perhaps even longer. All these unusual things make the bladder more likely to get infected (cystitis). It is important to drink lots of fluids and

to urinate frequently. Report any signs of burning and/or urgent
urination.

•Pains of various kinds may beset you. "Afterpains" are like labor
contractions, and they represent the same type of uterine muscular
activity. They usually last several days, are uncommon after the
first pregnancy, and are harder while you are nursing. Suckling is
nature's way of making your uterus come down in size, but it
increases the unpleasant uterine cramps. Particularly in the second
or third pregnancy, afterpains can be real attention-getters, but they
soon are gone.

•Your episiotomy is in a very sensitive place—between the vagina
and rectum—and can cause you some discomfort as you move
about. Speaking of moving, you may hope that your bowels do not
move again, ever! But they will, and all will stay together. In some
hospitals, you can take a sitz bath several times each day, and this
gives great local relief. Continue to do it at home. Your doctor has
probably ordered creams or other medications that will also give
you area relief. No matter what you do or don't do, the discomfort
gradually leaves completely, although for many months the
episiotomy site may throb somewhat during the first few days of
each period.

•Breast discomfort arrives about the time you are ready to go
home—or with today's abbreviated stays, a few days after you get
home. Your breasts become very congested, but not with milk.
That comes a day or so after the congestion. Whether or not
nursing is your goal, support your breasts with a good bra, but not
tightly, and use local heat or cold—whichever feels best. Milk
appears shortly after the congestion recedes. Breast infections are
unusual and do not appear until later. The symptoms are fever,
local breast redness, and pain. This is a doctor situation.

•As a result of the bearing down required of you, and because of the
local rectal dilation during labor, hemorrhoids are not unusual. As
in the earlier instructions on hemorrhoid care, avoid straining when
you move your bowels, be sure you are getting bulk in your diet or
with supplements, and use a stool softener if necessary. Your doctor
can provide local medications for pain relief. Your bowel function
should return promptly after delivery, unless elimination has always
been a problem for you. In that case, you should already have a
bowel program.

The Blues

We have already talked about "baby blues," and you know that it can happen to you no matter how happy you are and how well things seem to be going. Even in your most joyous moments you may burst out crying. But don't despair; it is transient and will soon be gone. In a few instances (less than 15 percent), postpartum depression (PPD) becomes a real monster and must be dealt with early on. This is most likely to affect those mothers who have a history of depression or who became significantly depressed at some point earlier in their pregnancy. Fortunately, these depressions will respond to modern medications and counseling. Many support groups are available—by phone or mail and on the Internet. Contact, for example, Depression After Delivery (DAD) at (800) 944–4773 or online at www.behavenet.com/dadinc. AOL offers a PPD message board and a weekly support group on Wednesdays at 9:00 P.M. EST ("Topic Chatroom" under MOMS Online).

Hygiene

Your personal hygiene need not change much after a vaginal delivery, except that you cannot wear tampons (I don't think you would want to anyway) and you cannot douche. Otherwise, you may shower and wash your hair and also take tub baths. Sometimes, as we already noted, sitting in the tub a spell brings considerable relief to that weary, painful area. Most hospitals provide facilities to do such cleansing, and you will feel better for it—if you are there long enough!

After a Section

You are now both postoperative and postpartum. You are likely to recover a little more slowly after a section, and the feelings are different than they are after a vaginal delivery. The first hospital day you will be up, but you will enjoy your bed very much. You may be carrying an in-dwelling bladder catheter that will probably be removed that first day. You may be fed intravenously for a while, but light oral feedings may be offered. There is more discomfort at the operative site, and you are given somewhat stronger pain relief. On the other hand, the anesthesiologist may have left your epidural catheter in place for the first day, and pain control may be continued by that route. Generally, by the second day all catheters have been removed and you are encouraged to be up and move about more actively. Oral feedings have been established, and you will progress to a full diet as rapidly as you can tolerate hospital food—or someone else's cooking if you are going home, and you probably are. The next few days are made memorable to you by copious gas, which collects in your colon and thunderously awaits your recovering ability to expel it. This usually happens when there are visitors in the house! At any rate, you will be glad to see and hear the last of it—and perhaps of your guests as well.

You will require more rest and more help at home than you would after a vaginal delivery. Remember—you are postoperative. While recovery from an uncomplicated section is usually quite rapid, you still must pace yourself. If your doctor does not object, you may shower as soon as you wish—unless you have some sutures and clips that require an abdominal dressing. Ask.

More Hospital Chores

•Your doctor or an associate or a nurse-practitioner will see you each day that you stay. Should you have a pediatrician, he or she will also see you daily. It may be hard to know what questions to ask, but don't hesitate to ask anything of anyone. This is particularly true about topics such as nursing and, should you have a son, circumcision (see next section).

•If you are Rh-negative, be sure that your vaccination program is carried out if it is deemed necessary. This is almost never overlooked in any hospital setting, but it is worth double-checking.

•If you are not already immune to German measles, now is a good time to be vaccinated. All you have to do is keep from getting pregnant for the next 60 days! You've survived greater challenges than that.

Circumcision—The Unkindest Cut?

Mutilation of both male and female external genital organs has been conducted as long as recorded history—and maybe even longer. The external genitals of little girls are still being carved upon in certain cultures, and one goal of the United Nations Health Organization is to end this barbarous practice everywhere. Similarly, little boys' external genitals have been massively mutilated in past (and some present) societies, and circumcision—the removal of the penis foreskin—is considered by many to be simply an extension and continuation of that mutilation.

Those who support the continuation of this procedure, however, argue:

•Virtually all penis cancer occurs in uncircumcised males.

•The incidence of recurrent herpes virus lesions and other STDs is reduced in circumcised males.

•There is no risk of phimosis (stricture of the foreskin) and resultant damage to the upper urinary system.

•The risk of cancer of the cervix is greater among women with uncircumcised male partners.

•Prostate cancer is more common in uncircumcised males.

Those who oppose the procedure argue:

•The operation is dangerous. One in 1,000 bleed, one in 4,000 require sutures, and one in 15,000 require plastic repair surgery.

•The operation is painful—even with local anesthetics—and traumatizes the infant for several days thereafter.

•Sexual gratification may be reduced in later years.

•Circumcision represents a barbarous, ritualistic carryover from times best forgotten.

So—scanning all these pros and cons, how can you make an informed and proper decision?

You can't. Virtually no one can make a dispassionate decision, because we are all still wrapped in and warped by generational and cultural dogma—the same being true of your doctors and attendants. There is firm evidence that circumcision does what both its proponents and opponents say it does—and on that note, I will close this discussion.

Some Things to Do at Home

Unfortunately, because of a repeated distortion of our cultural patterns, and because of the impact of all media advertising, we tend to get our priorities in marriage reversed. Daily we are reminded that our children—bonding with them, their education, health, and security—come first. Next comes a clean kitchen and the proper selection of detergents and coffee. After all this comes social, school, religious, and cultural responsibilities, including the PTA, the Little League, the sale of Girl Scout cookies, and the ERA. After that comes your makeup, the length of your hem, and the state of your cooking and your Jane Fonda warm-ups. And last, unless I've forgotten something else of greater importance, your husband or your mate and your relationship with him.

The truth, of course, is that the most important single thing in your life, other than your own identity, self-esteem, and growth as an individual, is your relationship with him—both socially and sexually. If your relationship together doesn't come first, nothing else, in the long run, will be meaningful and satisfactory for either of you. We are apparently the sexiest society going. But once we start living together and raising a family, it all seems to cease. Whoever saw a husband and wife kiss on a TV commercial? Really kiss? But this is life, not TV, so don't just keep him around for sentimental reasons. Hug him and talk to him!

Coming home from the hospital is a very critical time. I hope someone has impressed this upon you. To begin with, you are not as strong as you thought you were when you left the hospital, and you have a new, 24-hour, demanding, if lovable and loving responsibility—and unlike in British movies, you have no nanny to hand the baby back to after feeding time. And, for that matter, no nanny to bring food to you or to make your bed or clean your home. Moreover, your mate may not easily adjust to sharing you and your love with this new love, particularly if he or she is the firstborn. You understand that he loves you and that he loves the baby, but he is perhaps jealous of the baby's position in your loving order. Don't neglect each other.

Equally important, you may be somewhat depressed because of the "baby blues." That we have talked about. Although this is usually a mild complaint, it is a contributing factor at this uncertain time.

Then, as a final blow, friends or relatives may be ever-present, suggesting, interfering, confusing you. They are usually a pleasant and helpful lot, but they have a tendency to overstay. You may soon feel that *you* had an operation and *they* had a baby.

In view of all these things, a good plan for the early days at home would be as follows: Unless you dwell in a mansion and are accustomed to servants, don't have anybody living in except your husband. Get your help from him. You may need extra day help with cleaning, shopping, and so on, but have as little as possible. Your mother or his mother may wish to come and help, but even if it is necessary and they do, as soon as possible try to make it on your own. Don't have visitors unless you want them. Get your advice from your doctor. As soon as you are able, step out with your main man—without your baby—and keep your private life going. You are not a slave, and it was never intended that you spend the rest of your days and nights cooped up in a house or an apartment doing the same dull things over and over again. That leads to "cabin fever," and cabin fever leads to trouble. Remember that!

Make your baby feel secure and loved when you are together, but learn to leave him or her with others for short periods of time. After all, at 18 or so—if you're lucky—this loving child is going to shake your hand, say, "Thanks a lot for everything," and leave. If you have made a pattern of devoting your entire life to that child, you will find yourself with 30 or 40 years left over to share with no one. This is good advice.

It is very important in parenting to make all your children feel wanted and loved. Very important. But it does not require your undivided 24-hour attention to impart that feeling to them. Give them their fair share of quality time. Then take off.

Your family and relatives may not agree—but take a close look at their experience.

Activities

It is difficult to say exactly how active any individual mother can be when she gets home. There is a tremendous variation in energy level and in personal and family responsibilities. You probably find that you tire more easily than you might expect, and you must key your activities to this fact. Since you are to be up at night for some weeks to come, try to establish an afternoon sleep period each day. If you continually push yourself too hard, you only delay your complete recovery.

Taking stairs and going outside are not a problem—unless they are a problem! Too many stairs and weather that is too hot, too cold, or too wet when you do get out can be problems. If you are willing to face traffic, there is no reason you cannot go for an automobile ride whenever you want. You may drive the car yourself when you feel steady enough—except after a section. When you are recovering from a section, you must get cleared by your obstetrician to be certain wound healing has moved along okay. Buckle up everybody.

Although your stomach muscles and skin have been stretched greatly by pregnancy and are loose and flabby, they are yours to keep. For the sake of your posture, your back, and your self-esteem, you need to get these stretched straps toned again as soon as you can. You may begin exercising at any time, even while you are still in the hospital, and even if you have had a cesarean section. The trouble is—and you soon find this out—there is very little time and energy left over for formal exercises. But ask the physical therapist in the hospital to demonstrate a series of exercises—if you are there long enough. Otherwise, there are any number of tapes, videos, and books on the subject. Just be sure you follow a program specifically recommended for the postpartum period. The rest is up to you.

One solution to the exercise problem is to become involved in some outdoor sport activity, weather permitting. You may choose swimming, tennis, or golf, all of which are ready for you as soon as you are ready for them. Bicycling and horseback riding are ready for you whenever your bottom or your incision is ready. More aggressive activities, such as water skiing, should be delayed three or four weeks, but the key is to *get out and get active* in something that is interesting and exercise those flabby muscles. Aerobics—either a video, as suggested, or a class—provides an excellent way to get started in this program. When there is time!

Hygiene

As you have seen, hospital routines allow you to shower, bathe, and wash your hair anytime you wish—again, except for sections. Moreover, following a vaginal delivery, you are encouraged to take sitz baths to help heal your episiotomy. When you get home, instead of taking a sitz bath, just go ahead and take a full tub bath, which is both cleansing and healing. You may also, of course, shower and shampoo. But if you shower rather than bathe, be sure your perineum, the area of your episiotomy, between the vagina and rectum, is kept scrupulously clean. You will continue to have a heavy vaginal discharge (lochia), which gradually subsides during the first month at home. Originally blood-tinged, this discharge gradually becomes more and more yellowish and eventually disappears. Once the secretion is light enough and the perineum has healed sufficiently, you may use a tampon instead of an external pad. You can use a tampon anytime after a cesarean section, if it is agreeable with your physician. If you nurse, you may have a light vaginal discharge for a longer period of time and, of course, may not have menstrual periods at all. In the event of a sudden heavy increase in the amount of blood in your lochia, call your doctor. Generally speaking, you will have your first menstrual period (provided you are not nursing) somewhere during the first four to eight weeks after delivery. It is all right to use birth control pills as a form of contraception if you are not nursing. You may begin them while you are in the hospital. If you are nursing, there is a progestin-only birth control pill that is effective and apparently safe.

Medications

Continue to take your vitamin supplements for several months after you deliver, and if you are nursing, continue the supplements at least until your baby is weaned. You may require no other medication except an occasional laxative. However, if you need something for pain or for the blues, your doctor will order it for you—being aware that you may be nursing. Perhaps you are on other medications for certain problems that predated your pregnancy or developed while you were pregnant. You will most certainly receive specific instructions about their continuing use. If you are nursing, do not start any new medication on your own. Mother's milk passes not only nutrients on to your baby but almost everything running around in your bloodstream.

The Call to Arms

Generally speaking, before you have been home too long, *somebody* will think of sex again, and suddenly a great amount of activity and interest is generated in that direction. Although your episiotomy will have healed within a few weeks, there is often enough residual discomfort to make vaginal penetration uncomfortable. It is a good idea to avoid this degree of sexual activity until after your first office visit, but not many people do! Remember, though, you may be fertile and you do not want to make your first postpartum visit your first prenatal visit. You may make all kinds of love without vaginal penetration anytime you want to.

Postpartum Check

While you are still in the hospital after delivery, it is a good idea to call your doctor's office and make arrangements for your first postpartum examination, which used to be about six weeks after you delivered but now may take place as early as two weeks, depending upon your doctor's instructions. By the time of this first visit, you are recovered sufficiently so that the doctor can examine you internally to make sure that your body has healed and the uterus is returning to normal size, shape, and position. Also at this time you want to discuss the various methods of birth control, provided you are not already on oral contraceptives (OCs), and provided that you wish to avoid populating the world. The alternatives are looked at in the next section. If a Pap smear is due, it will be taken at that time; if not, your doctor will be able to tell you when you must return for it. This is probably the most important single test a woman has available to her today. If for no other reason than obtaining your Pap smear, a postpartum visit is of fundamental importance because it continues and reinforces the concept of a regular checkup. If you have any trouble with your breasts or if you are nursing, your doctor may want to examine your breasts, as he or she undoubtedly will during your annual checkup—along with your mammogram if you are of that age.

Returning to the Workaday World

In today's environment, you will probably either want or need to return to your former employment. Most organizations now have specific maternity leave policies; generally you can return to work with your position and seniority intact. The average leave time has been six weeks after the actual date of delivery, but there are now tremendous variations: Longer leave periods are now often available. The magazine *Working Mother* publishes an annual report on this issue along with a list of the 100 best companies in terms of employee care. If your delivery has been complicated or your baby has a significant health problem, you may need extended leave until all is stable at home. Your doctor can see to it that the proper information reaches your employer. The Federal Family Leave Act makes all this easier to arrange. Incidentally, day care, a massive problem today, is often provided by major employers.

Here are some further points about working after delivery.

- A part-time or compressed-time job or a job-sharing relationship may work for you. Moreover, it is becoming increasingly popular to allow computer-linked work to be done at home. Everything but the company rest rooms seems to be computer-linked today.

- Paternity leave is becoming more common and more acceptable at corporate levels. Some men take off a year to share the intimate work of parenting an infant. Again, federal legislation is making this easier to accomplish.

- It is generally good for you to get back to your work environment, particularly if you enjoy what you do and the people you work with. It gets you out of the house and prevents cabin fever. Moreover, it is very important that you keep your own life going, and this is a good, rewarding way to start.

- Obviously *some* jobs are more physical than others. Thus, a forklift operator, a forest ranger, a secretary, a floor duty nurse, and a commercial airline pilot all must meet different requirements before returning to their duties after childbirth.

- Studies show that periods of separation from your child are not in the least detrimental to your relationship with each other or to the child's emotional growth and security—provided, of course, that you do spend plenty of quality time together and continue to bond.

You are now fulfilling many roles: parent, partner, worker, house-keeper, cook, and lover. This is a difficult assignment, and you will need and deserve help from that other partner in order to fulfill all these roles. Thus, if it's Saturday night at eleven o'clock, and you have had a rough week at the office (worker), managed an aggressive, active, fussy child all day (parent), and in the meantime did the week's laundry (housekeeper) and took care of the weekend's menu (cook), you don't have much reserve left if the call to arms should come (lover). So each must share the wealth and the work.

Try to resolve your personal conflicts about work and what it means to your relationship with your child before you return to work. Get your priorities listed and in order. Carry them to work with you instead of guilt.

It is increasingly important in your personal life to be able to plan adequately for the growth and development of your family. At this point, you and/or your partner may begin to equate self-control with birth control. To this end, you may want to familiarize yourself with the most common acceptable forms of personal family planning.

More Children?

There are many forms of birth control that you can consider.

The Pill

The original oral contraceptive was a sleeping pill. As time went on, it was replaced by *The Late, Late Show,* which was even less effective. Neither offered 24-hour protection, and a significant number of normal, healthy people make love at other times than bedtime. The market was there, and so, in the early 1950s, there became available "the pill." This pill—the *real* oral contraceptive—was a combination of hormones that incorporate some form of estrogen or estrogen-like substance and a progestin (a progesterone-like substance), estrogen and progesterone being the two female hormones. These pills had the almost unfailing ability to prevent ovulation. They provided, therefore, almost 100 percent pregnancy protection.

The early pills were of a much higher dose range than those marketed today, and so many side effects were noted. Weight gain, fluid retention, headaches, absence of periods, breast tenderness, and more were all very common problems associated with the pill. Very dangerous complications such as intravascular clotting with embolism formation and serious liver tumors were reported often enough to give both the doctor and patient considerable concern. These events are extremely rare today, since we are into the third-generation pill—in a much lower, yet still protective, dose range. Although there are still unwanted side effects such as weight gain, headaches, acne, and so forth, generally a formula can be found that is agreeable and the dangerous complications have become extremely remote.

Let's look at the modern low-dose pill and its risks and benefits.

- •The benefits:
  - virtually 100 percent effective birth control
  - less menstrual cramping
  - shorter periods, therefore less blood loss and less anemia
  - fewer cases of benign breast disease—some 25,000 fewer annual breast biopsies
  - less ovarian cyst formation
  - fewer ectopic pregnancies

fewer pelvic infections from sexually transmitted disease
less risk of ovarian and uterine cancer in later years
less rheumatoid arthritis risk

•The risks:
cancer of the breast—no clear risk as yet established (There may
  be a slight risk after long-term use, but the tumors are less
  aggressive, with an excellent arrest rate.)
intravascular clotting (rare)
side effects such as headaches, amenorrhea, hypertension, and
  weight gain (all unusual with the third-generation pill)

As times goes on, the relative safety of the low-dose pills becomes
more clearly established—so much so that these pills may now be taken
on into the forties, provided that the taker is also a nonsmoker and has
no contraindicating hypertensive cardiovascular disorder. As long as serious side effects do not occur, the pill may be used without interruption
for many years of reproductive life and as a vehicle to carry you through
the early menopausal years with the same generous protection and the
same slight risks. As mentioned earlier, some pure progestin pills are considered safe to use while nursing and, further, may be safe to use if you
have a history of intravascular clotting. You will need help here to determine the safety of these agents.

The IUD

Some of us feel that if you're not taking oral contraceptive pills you are
simply taking chances. However, there are a number of plastic or plas-
tic/metal intrauterine devices—IUDs—that can be inserted into the uterus
and left there, and they are very effective methods of birth control. No
one really knows for sure how IUDs work, but it is assumed that they
prevent the implantation of a fertilized ovum into the uterine wall. Such
devices are usually inserted just before the end of a menstrual flow, and
sometimes this insertion produces discomfort. They are difficult to place
in women who have not had children, but it can be done with care.

IUDs are not 100 percent effective. Of pregnancies that do take place,
most occur in the first year after insertion. The rate of pregnancy is
around 2 percent the first year, decreasing each year thereafter.
Occasionally it is necessary to remove an IUD because of side effects,
such as prolonged and heavy bleeding both during and between periods,
severe cramping, or recurrent infection. A plastic IUD may be left in
place indefinitely if there are no local reactions. The copper and/or hormone IUDs must be replaced every few years. These devices are clearly
the most effective birth control agents after the pill. Some years ago one
particular IUD (no longer available) was accused of causing major repro-

ductive and health problems, but the IUDs on the market today have an excellent safety and birth control record.

The Rest

None of the other contraceptive devices compare to the pill or the IUD in preventing pregnancy.

Diaphragms, jellies, creams, foams, condoms (rubbers, sheaths, safes, balloons, whatever) are reasonably effective if used conscientiously. Often, in the heat of passion, they are forgotten. Condoms do have the advantage—a major advantage today—of helping to prevent the spread of sexually transmitted diseases.

Nursing is nature's contraception. Generally a nursing mother does not ovulate, and the longer she nurses, the longer she is unable to conceive. This is why, generations ago, women nursed until they could no longer stand the bites inflicted on their nipples by their "babies." However, ovulation *can* occur during nursing and therefore so can pregnancy. Remember, the progestin-only pill is a viable alternative.

Rhythm birth control is based upon the fact that ovulation pretty generally takes place at midcycle, about the 14th day of a 28-day cycle. A variety of signs—both local and general—herald ovulation, and there are various test kits available to help in its determination, a particularly important help in the presence of irregular cycles. When closely and religiously adhered to—and this means knowing your cycles and using your ovulation kit—rhythm provides reasonably effective birth control.

Speed Breeding

To all of you who are interested in populating the world, have no financial problems, and are not worried about increasing our risks of imminent extinction, you may plan your birth control in this general area, which includes: speedy withdrawal, douches, and hunches. Don't play any of these games.

Emergency Contraception

It happens. It not infrequently happens. For whatever reason or under whatever circumstance—unplanned, good, bad, average, thrilling, or disastrous—you have an unprotected sexual encounter—that is, birth control was not involved. Enter the emergency contraceptive pills.

These pills are just regular OCs taken in a modified way. The dose is usually four pills, which must be taken according to the directions and within 72 hours after the encounter. The sooner the better. They are very effective. Call at once—no later than the morning after.

Sterilization

Permanent and virtually perfect birth control is achieved by ligation of either the male vas deferens or the female fallopian tubes. Let's first consider ligation of the male vas.

- •Advantages of male sterilization:

    It can be done anytime, providing the operating physician is satisfied that the man is a responsible adult who is able to give his informed consent and wants no more children.

    It is a relatively safe, simple, quick procedure that can be done under local anesthesia. Vas ligation is therefore usually an office procedure, followed by only a few days' disability.

    It has no proven long- or short-term effects—except sterilization. Read on, though.

    Its effectiveness is very easy to prove: A negative sperm count indicates success.

- •Disadvantages of male sterilization:

    It is permanent. True, microsurgery can reconnect the tubes, but it is not always successful, and when vas ligation is done, it should be assumed that it is intended to be permanent. Is that a disadvantage? It is if you change your mind or your partner later in life.

    Other than the possible complications of any *minor* surgery, two side effects should be mentioned. There is some evidence that after vas ligation immune changes may occur that, in some men, can hasten the onset of arteriosclerosis (hardening of the arteries). The once-held position that vas ligation increases men's risk of prostate cancer is no longer tenable. As a final note, the act of sterilization may, in rare instances, induce psychological changes resulting in temporary impotence.

In women, bilateral tubal ligation has become a relatively simple procedure to arrange for and to accomplish. There are few legal or medical obstacles left to performing this minor surgery on mature consenting women. Frequently the tubes are tied through a very small incision immediately after delivery. If delivery is by cesarean section, then of course there is no need for any further incision. The tubes can be clipped, tied, sectioned, or removed at that time; it makes little difference how they are interrupted. Having your tubes tied at delivery usually requires that you spend no longer in the hospital than you normally would. The procedure is usually carried out through a very small incision just below the umbilicus. There are some situations, however, that make immediate tubal ligation unsafe after a vaginal delivery—a full stomach, for instance. Your doctor knows this and may do what is known as an interval sterilization—putting off surgery for 24–48 hours after delivery, or even until some months later.

Elective interval sterilization is now a relatively simple laparoscopic procedure commonly done without hospital admission, that is, as an outpatient. You are given a light general or local anesthetic, and a small hollow tube is inserted into your abdomen just below your navel. Your fallopian tubes are easily seen and localized and are then crushed, cauterized, or pulled through a small plastic ring or a clamp and pinched off completely. After a few hours of recovery, you go home. Very rarely, something can go wrong with this seemingly simple procedure, as it can with any operation. Therefore, you might, however unlikely it is, end up with a big incision in your abdomen, after several days in the hospital.

Another type of interval sterilization performed nowadays is called a minilap tubal ligation. This procedure avoids some of the problems associated with the umbilical type of procedure and is done through a small incision slightly below the pubic hairline. Each fallopian tube is grasped and a portion removed therefrom. This separates the ends completely from each other.

Here are some things to think about.

- •Advantages of female sterilization:
    It eliminates the need for birth control pills or any other devices.
    It is a permanent sterilization—but keep reading.
    It is almost foolproof.
    It has no sexual or other side effects that can be directly
        attributed to the procedure.
    It is relatively simple and very safe.
    The risk of ovarian cancer is reduced!

- •Disadvantages of female sterilization:
    It is permanent. As with male sterilization, there are
        microsurgical techniques to reverse tubal ligation, but such
        surgery is not always successful. So tubal ligation should be
        considered a permanent sterilization procedure.
    Fallopian tube ligation is not as simple as ligating the vas in a
        male. It is usually more expensive than a vas ligation (unless
        you have comprehensive insurance). Your insurance may not
        cover the procedure at all. You had better check first.
    It is not easy—as it is in the male—to test the success of the
        ligation.
    The regular failure rate may be as high as 2 percent, and there is
        also an increased risk that a subsequent pregnancy may be an
        ectopic one.

All sterilization procedures need to be preceded by adequate and thorough counseling that reveals the risks and benefits clearly.

The Last Pregnant Pauses

•What is the relative death risk of using oral contraceptives as compared to certain other risks in life? Well, the probability of death per year from oral contraceptive use is 1 in 63,000. Let's compare this to other risks:

Smoking	1 in 200
Driving	1 in 6,000
Sex (STDs)	1 in 50,000
Legal abortion	1 in 100,000 by 12th week
Legal abortion	1 in 10,000 after 16th week
Normal delivery	1 in 15,000

Source: *Contemporary OB/GYN* (December 1990)

•In 1952, Virginia Apgar, a pioneer neonatologist of immense stature, devised a quick system of assessing fetal well-being at and shortly after birth. The system, which carries her name, comprises five fetal signs (muscle tone, heart rate, color, respirations, and reflexes) taken at one minute and at five minutes. Her scoring system has been misused in recent years to indicate many neurological conditions on which it has no bearing. One of Dr. Apgar's last wishes was that her score be supplemented with a proper biochemical sampling of the fetal umbilical blood at birth.

•A survey conducted by the Kaiser Family Foundation of Menlo Park, California, revealed that most men (72 percent) and women (73 percent) felt that men did not participate enough in making sure that contraception is used. Men said they would try birth control pills (66 percent), long-acting shots (43 percent), or under-the-skin pellets (36 percent), but less than half the women questioned believed that men would actually do those things! (*Medical Economics: Obstetrics and Gynecology,* August 1997)

•Laboring and delivering in an upright, squatting, or sitting position is an instinctive practice dating back to the beginning of recorded obstetrical history. You might rightly wonder, then, at what point in time and for what reason the dorsal-recumbency (flat on your back in bed) position was adopted. Well, according to medical historians, sometime in the 17th century King Louis XIV of France made it known that he wished to observe his mistress giving birth. Thus, by royal edict, dorsal recumbency became the way to go. Moreover, as operative procedures and anesthesia became more common, so did the routine continuation of the supine position.

• Anthropological studies show that women laboring by themselves assume a variety of positions. Modern obstetrics has adopted this time-honored tradition and is more likely to let women labor in the position they find comfortable and helpful. And no king will be watching!

• In December 1927, a 24-year-old pregnant mother at full term was moving from Wisconsin to New York with her husband, who was testing his chances for a legal career in the big city. She was alone, and they were low on funds. From her place in Brooklyn Heights she could just see the clustered, exciting towers of lower Manhattan. She was unable to join the throng of happy Christmas shoppers because of her confinement and her purse. It was during these lonely days that she composed the following poem:

> O Thou, who maketh all things new,
> Who painteth pansies, and with sweetest breath,
> Hath kissed the petals of the folded rose
> And left them fragrant in their perfectness,
> Take Thou this new, wee babe
> Which throbs so gently 'neath
> its mother's heart
> Protect it in Thy deep enfolding love
> And guide it as it grows a child complete,
> Ready to meet the lessons of Thy glowing world
> With eager mind and quick truth-seeking eye
> Let it know Thee that it may someday share
> Thy wondrous power and everlasting peace,
> That it may see Thy gentleness and love,
> Thy quick forgiveness, tender, merciful,
> And when my babe is perfect at Thy side,
> Give it to me to keep a while for Thee,

And guide me through this holiest of trusts
That I may daily worthy of it be.

Soon after, this mother delivered a son who grew to be a noted American columnist and who found this poem some 55 years later in his mother's personal papers.

Diary

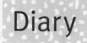

(My Tenth Month)

At last!

My thoughts and feelings_____

_____

_____

_____

_____

_____

_____

MY DELIVERY

Date_____

Where_____

_____

My companion(s)_____

_____

_____

Times

In hospital_____

Labor_____

Delivered_____

_____

Vaginal birth or cesarean_____

_____

_____

Anesthetic_____

_____

Anesthesiologist or anesthetist present_____

_____

Baby

Sex_____

Weight_____

Apgar at one minute_____

Apgar at five minutes_____

Cord blood saved_____

Special circumstances_____

_____

_____

_____

Delivered by_____

Assistant(s)_____

_____

My personal notes about my labor and delivery_____

_____

_____

_____

_____

_____

_____

_____

_____

_____

_____

_____

_____

_____

_____

Appendix: Obstetrical Technology

Obstetrical technology is growing at an incredible pace. This appendix is devoted to a brief encounter with most of the new techniques, tests, devices, and procedures involved in the present-day delivery of obstetrical care. Your own doctor will also be aware of when and how these programs change. And change they will!

Genetics

All of us have a genetic code that endows us with our unalterable, inherited characteristics. Of all the magic and mystery that enshroud procreation and life, none surpasses the binding of the total and absolutely necessary coded material into a single sperm head and a single ovum, which then unite with each other to unravel that fantastic code and weave, on an embryo's magic loom, a new body, mind, and spirit with the characteristics—good, bad, indifferent, and so-so—of both parents and a heavenly host of ancestors and progenitors.

Geneticists found that in each human cell there are 46 chromosomes: 22 pairs of autosomes and 2 sex chromosomes. Women have two X sex chromosomes (XX) and men an X and a Y sex chromosome (XY). The female's two Xs actually outweigh the male's XY and also carry more information. Let me point out, however, that most often, of the female's two Xs, only one is working; the other is lying at the bottom of each cell, apparently doing nothing. We can see this phenomenon under the microscope. The nonworking X chromosome is called a Barr body (after the scientist who discovered the phenomenon); its presence (or absence) helps us in the study of certain genetic and infertility problems.

Of the 46 paired chromosomes in each cell, one member of each pair comes from the sperm, one from the ovum. (The split of the paired chromosomes occurs just as the egg and sperm mature.) Since half of the sperm contain X sex chromosomes and half contain Y, and since all ova contain only one X, then it follows that the male determines the sex.

Each chromosome contains a number of stations of dots, called genes, and these, too, are paired: Some genes are "dominant" and some "recessive," and recessives "give" to the dominant gene. Thus, brown eyes (BB) dominate blue eyes (bb), and a union of these two traits would always produce a brown-eyed child (almost always anyway). Although oversimplified, that is the basic principle involved in dominant and recessive genes and their function.

The task of mapping the entire human system of genes—up to 85,000 in number—has now been undertaken. Called the Human Genome Project, we have already located about 16,000 genes, and many have already been of clinical use. The worldwide mapping project should be completed very early in the next millennium—no later than the year 2005. As the mapping unfolds, more and more help will be provided to clinicians and to their patients.

It is important to know that chromosomes can be damaged by toxic substances, heat (but not cold—one can freeze and preserve sperm, eggs, and embryos with safety), X-rays, age, and certain other conditions. It is also important to know that most defective embryos are scanned and destroyed by nature, either by early miscarriage or by initial failure to even imbed in the uterine lining. *Well over 25 percent of all conceptions end up this way.*

Chromosomal abnormalities increase regularly and significantly with maternal age. Thus, at age 25, the frequency of chromosomal abnormality is 1 in 476, while at 43 it has risen to 1 in 31. Paternal age is also a factor, but less so than maternal age.

Genetic Tests Available Today

- **Maternal serum alpha-fetoprotein (MSAFP)** screening. This test is really a screen for potentially incomplete fetal neural tube closure (spina bifida, for instance) rather than a direct genetic test. It is usually performed during the 15th week of pregnancy. Read more about it further on. As far as genetics is concerned, it is just a screening procedure.

- **Ultrasound** in early pregnancy may produce results that suggest a need for direct genetic testing.

•**Amniocentesis.** For genetic screening, this procedure is carried out at 16–17 weeks as a rule. Read about it in detail in a moment.

•**Chorionic villi sampling (CVS).** Samples of placental tissue are sucked away through the cervix—usually at 10–12 weeks. Read about it also in a moment.

•**Maternal blood analysis.** A relative newcomer. Special procedures separate the fetal blood cells circulating in the maternal blood. These separated cells are then submitted for DNA testing, which isolates chromosomes X, Y, 21, 18, and 13. These five chromosomes contain 95 percent of all fetal genetic abnormalities. In this regard, it falls 5 percent short of CVS and amniocentesis.

•**Cervical washings.** This procedure—also a new newcomer— involves running a catheter through the cervical canal and washing out fetal/placental cells that have been shed and come to rest just above the cervix. These cells are then identified as of fetal origin and are subjected to analysis. There is, as yet, very little to report about this new technique.

Types of Genetic Disorders

Dominant. Because the gene is dominant, only one parent has to carry the defective gene. Achondroplastic dwarfs who have short arms and legs are an example of this type of disorder.

Recessive. Such disorders require that both parents supply the abnormal gene. The most striking example is muscular dystrophy, which almost always occurs in white people of northern European descent. Other examples are sickle cell anemia, which affects mainly African Americans; Tay-Sachs disease, which affects Ashkenazi Jews; and beta-thalassemia, a type of anemia found usually in persons of middle Mediterranean descent.

Sex-linked disorders. Sex-linked problems are usually recessive gene disorders found on the X (thus sex) chromosome. Hemophilia is the most common example.

Chromosomal disorders. These inherited conditions involve the movement (translocation) and absence or shortening of whole portions of chromosomes. Down's syndrome falls into this category.

Multiple disorders. We mentioned earlier that environmental problems can induce genetic mutations and other chromosomal abnormalities. Chernobyl, Hiroshima, and Love Canal are glaring examples, but there are many less striking instances all around us. These external factors work their will on a vulnerable gene to produce the congenital anomaly. Most commonly, heart defects and neural tube defects (spina bifida, for example) are produced.

Prenatal Genetic Counseling

All of these congenital disorders may be diagnosed prenatally, using various combinations of maternal blood tests, amniocentesis, chorionic villi sampling, and ultrasound.

Who should have prenatal genetic counseling?

- couples with a familial or racial history of an inherited disorder

- couples who already have a genetically abnormal child

- mothers in their late thirties or older

- couples who have sustained multiple miscarriages or fetal losses and stillbirths

Some final genetic points:

- There are over 1,200 full-time genetic counselors in this country. Their increasing availability makes it easier for obstetricians to involve them in your genetic investigation.

- Almost 130 different genetic disorders can now be identified. While it is true that many of them are rare, at least 10 of them are relatively common disorders.

- Progress in the Human Genome Project is now so rapid that most physicians cannot possibly stay current with what is being found. A website is now being established to help overcome this informational lag.

Amniocentesis

As the word indicates, *amniocentesis* is the removal of amniotic fluid from the amniotic sac. The fetus is enclosed in two sacs, the more proximate one being called the amniotic sac or membrane. Within its confines, besides the fetus, is a clear liquid appropriately called the amniotic fluid, which increases from 80 cc's (2¾ oz) at 12 weeks to as much as 1,500 cc's (1½ qt) at term. There may be too much fluid (polyhydramnios) or too little (oligohydramnios); such extremes usually, but not always, signify a fetal disturbance or a structural abnormality.

Water, which accounts for 98 percent of the fluid, is renewed about every three hours, while other components (electrolytes, proteins, and so on) change at a slower pace. This renewal phenomenon indicates that an amniotic circulation must exist, and indeed it does, although the mechanism is not altogether clear. At term an infant swallows about 450 cc's of amniotic fluid every 24 hours and quite regularly empties its bladder back into the amniotic sac. But these basic exchanges are insufficient to account for the total renewal of all amniotic elements. Other maternal-fetal circulatory and exchange mechanisms are obviously involved, but as yet they are not completely understood.

Amniotic fluid protects the fetus by providing constant temperature and pressure, plus a shock-absorbing environment that allows free body movement and growth. There are undoubtedly many other amniotic fluid functions that are unknown. The fluid also contains some fetal debris, traces of meconium (a forerunner of stools) from the rectum, and lanugo (soft downy body hair), as well as surface fetal skin cells that regularly fall away as new skin cells come to the surface. Finally, there are chemical substances circulating in the amniotic fluid. These substances are under constant study, and some are now used in a variety of tests to indicate fetal well-being, growth, and development and to help identify certain inherited problems such as sickle cell anemia.

For our purposes, amniocentesis is almost always accomplished by means of a transabdominal (through the maternal skin, abdominal wall, and uterus) needle puncture. There are several particular times in pregnancy that this procedure is brought into use for analysis.

As we have seen, genetic amniocentesis is employed during or close to the 15th week of pregnancy. Carefully guided by ultrasound, and with the mother under local anesthesia, a needle is inserted through the abdomen and uterus into the amniotic sac, and a measured amount of fluid is withdrawn. Some of this is used for certain chemical tests (a true alpha-fetoprotein or AFP test, for instance, which is more accurate than the usual maternal blood test). Most of the fluid, however, ends up being cultured so that the fetal skin cells within it may grow and be harvested in two or three weeks. Cells rarely fail to grow—but it can happen, and a repeat amniocentesis may be necessary. This can be a real problem with amniocentesis because, when cultures fail, we have lost several weeks and must start again. We are then into the fourth month of pregnancy and still awaiting a diagnosis.

When cellular growth is satisfactory, chemical agents are used to enlarge the fetal cell nucleus and geneticists then study them under very high magnification. Chromosomal analysis thus obtained is very accurate and allows—whether important to the parents or not—absolute prediction of the fetal sex.

The 15th week is generally chosen for two reasons. First, before that time it is difficult to obtain a sufficient amount of amniotic fluid, and second, as noted, any delay beyond 15 weeks makes a potential therapeutic abortion more difficult and more emotionally traumatic.

Early Amniocentesis Problems

•**Failure.** There are a number of reasons for this:

Insufficient amniotic fluid prevents the operator from either establishing contact with the amniotic sac or withdrawing enough fluid for analysis.

The placenta may be directly in the way and prevent entrance into the amniotic sac.

Maternal obesity may prevent needle penetration of sufficient depth into the abdomen.

•**Spontaneous abortion.** Although miscarriage does follow some amniocentesis procedures, the rate of occurrence is less than 1 percent—a lower figure than one would expect in a similar population of pregnant women not having any procedure done at all.

•**Rh sensitization.** Minute amounts of fetal blood *may* escape into the maternal circulation. In certain cases, a very few fetal red blood cells can produce an Rh interaction in the blood of the mother if she is Rh-negative and the fetus is Rh-positive. Since the fetal blood type is unknown, all Rh-negative women are immediately vaccinated with the Rh immune globulin after amniocentesis, and revaccinated with the same Rh vaccine at 28 weeks. Again, this is done even though the fetal Rh type is still unknown. There are no serious risks in giving the vaccine, but there are real risks in not giving it.

Some Further Amniocentesis Facts

•The reports that you anxiously await are generally available in three to four weeks, and you should be contacted immediately. The analysis involves alpha-fetoprotein testing for neural tube defects plus chromosomal culture and eventual analysis. The culturing is what takes time.

•The costs of amniocentesis, at this writing, vary in different locations across the United States from $1,000 to $1,500; the procedure is often covered by insurance. In some countries (Canada, for example), the national health plan will pick up the tab.

•The accuracy is virtually 100 percent, and a genetic abnormality is discovered in 3–5 percent of the pregnancies tested.

•Genetic counseling is available at all tertiary maternity care centers (see page 301) and in certain other locations. Your doctor is familiar with the center closest to you. Also, as noted earlier, there are increasing numbers of medical geneticists in practice everywhere.

Amniocentesis in Late Pregnancy

Amniocentesis becomes progressively *easier* as pregnancy advances (because there is more amniotic fluid), and it has been found to be of great value in later pregnancy for:

- •**Evaluation of fetal lung maturity.** There are many reasons why lung maturity is an important piece of information to have before contemplating an early delivery. Amniotic fluid reveals evidence of this in a variety of biochemical tests.

- •**Determination of fetal well-being.** In circumstances in which a child approaching term may be in jeopardy, such as with a diabetic mother or if intrauterine growth retardation (IUGR) or Rh incompatibility is suspected, amniotic fluid is a key source of information in the establishment of fetal well-being.

- •**Premature rupture of the membrane (PROM).** In the event that rupture may have taken place and cannot be simply detected by other means, the insertion of dye into the amniotic fluid helps to determine the integrity of the fetal sac. Dye found later in the vagina is proof of rupture.

- •**Culturing.** When the doctor suspects that an infection has developed in the fetal amniotic sac, fluid can be withdrawn for culturing purposes.

Chorionic Villi Sampling

This genetic sampling technique has long been used in other countries but is relatively new in the United States. After a proper period of experimental testing and application, it has now been proven reliable, accurate, and reasonably safe. It is therefore finding widespread use in this country, sometimes supplanting genetic amniocentesis at some centers.

The chorionic villi sampling technique is based on the fact that chorionic villi, the fetal tissue destined to form the placenta, completely surrounds the fetal sac in early pregnancy—somewhat like the fuzzy yellow covering of a new tennis ball. It is thus reasonably accessible for study in the very early weeks. Samples of these fetal tissues can be obtained either through the cervix or transabdominally, using ultrasound as a guide.

•Advantages
>Because the procedure can be done earlier in pregnancy (10–12
   weeks) than can amniocentesis, diagnosis can be made sooner
   and the pregnancy terminated more easily if that should be
   indicated.
>The laboratory results are obtained within a few days—once
   again accelerating the diagnosis time.
>It is somewhat less hazardous to the mother.
>It is more economical.

•Disadvantages
>Failure to achieve sufficient samples sometimes occurs.
>There is a slightly greater risk of abortion following the
   procedure than with amniocentesis.
>Accidental sampling of maternal tissue may produce false results.
>CVS will not detect neural tube defects as will amniocentesis.
   Therefore, MSAFP testing is still important. CVS also misses
   the fragile X syndrome—the most common cause of sex-
   linked inherited mental retardation. Otherwise, it is
   diagnostically faultless.
>It has been blamed for reduction in fetal limbs by several
   investigators, but recent work refutes most of these claims.
   This complication has apparently been related to very early
   CVS. Therefore, although the procedure can technically be
   accomplished well before ten weeks, it is not recommended to
   do so.

Chorionic villi samples are analyzed to determine the chromosomal,
enzymatic, and DNA status of the fetus. Unlike amniotic fluid, alpha-
fetoprotein testing cannot be done on chorionic villi samples, and that is
why neural tube defects go undetected.

DNA analysis is the study of desoxyribonucleic acid (DNA). These
coiled strands of nucleic acids are the substance of our genes and therefore the source of all that we are.

Alpha-Fetoprotein Test (AFP)

This test, which you now know is routinely done in early amniocentesis
procedures, can also be performed, with less precision, on maternal
blood serum (MSAFP) at about 14–15 weeks of pregnancy. By that time,
AFP should have almost disappeared from the fetal and therefore the
maternal circulation, since the fetal neural tube and the spinal canal,
where the fluid originates, should now be closed. Obstetricians are now
doing MSAFP tests on mothers routinely during the 14–15th week of

pregnancy. An abnormally high level may indicate that closure of the neural tube has not taken place. Thus, an ultrasound becomes vital to determine where the spinal defect may be. The problem could be anything from a mild spina bifida to an anencephalic (headless) infant—a dreadful deformity, incompatible with life. An abnormally elevated test may also indicate the pregnancy is not as far along as had been determined. Accurate dating then becomes very important.

Recent evidence shows that very low values of the MSAFP test in early pregnancy may indicate the presence of Down's syndrome.

Ultrasound

The advent of present-day reliable ultrasound techniques in obstetrics has had an impact on the American lifestyle, economy, and society equivalent to that of the advent of the automobile or electricity at the turn of the century. It is difficult to comprehend the magnitude of the obstetrical information this procedure has spawned. Ultrasound provides us with very reliable, detailed intrauterine evidence of the evolution of an embryo to a fetus to an infant as pregnancy advances to full term and the moment of delivery. Moreover—and of infinite importance—it is a procedure that is safe, practical, and almost universally available.

As the name implies, ultrasound is simply sound waves that have been machine-generated at a frequency of such magnitude that they cannot be heard. These very small, high-frequency waves can penetrate our bodies and bounce back from whatever they strike. The denser the tissue or organ, the greater the bounceback. That principle is what generates

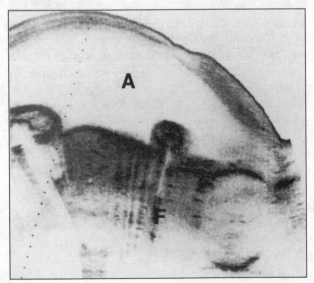

Here is an ultrasound of hydramnios. (see appendix). The white area (A) is amniotic fluid in very excessive amounts. The condition is usually associated with fetal developmental disorders.

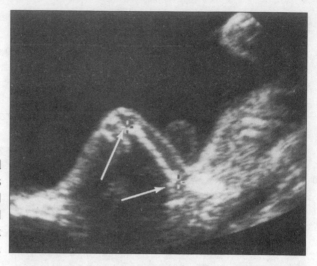

An unusually clear fetal profile. The femur is being measured between the arrows and indicates a 21-week fetus.

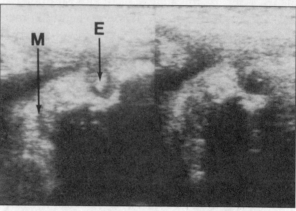

A baby's face with the eye (E) closed in one frame (left) and open in the other. The mouth (M) is clearly seen. Is it smiling?

the image that we see. As technology improves, so do the images—often even computer-enhanced to provide us with very clear pictures.

Generally speaking, *real-time* ultrasound is used most often now in obstetrical examinations—that is, what you see on the screen is what is actually going on right then. Although what is on the screen is not frozen into a photo, photos can be made at any point and preserved. Very early pregnancy ultrasounds may be done transvaginally with a safe, painless, and sterile transducer, while later procedures are done transabdominally.

Here are some examples of the use of ultrasound in obstetrics:

•**Monitoring of the fetal heart.** The fetal heart can be seen beating beginning at the seventh to eighth week of pregnancy—although very high-resolution ultrasound can see a cardiac tube pulsating as early as six weeks into the pregnancy! The absence of a heartbeat much after eight weeks generally indicates serious fetal problems.

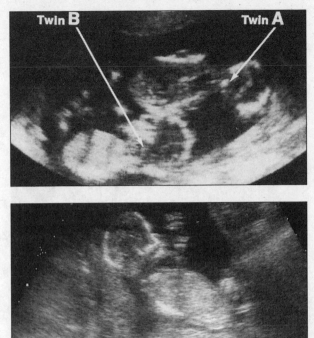

A set of 15-week twins, looking like two bowling pins lying side by side.

A 14-week fetus waving.

So if the examination is repeated a few days or a week later and still no heart activity is seen, we generally consider this fact to be absolute evidence of fetal demise. This information is of real value both to mother and to doctor. It prevents the prolonged, agonizing wait for a sure sign that something had gone wrong, as we often used to have to endure. So while it is rare and discouraging not to have a visible heartbeat by at least the ninth week, it is extremely reassuring to see it.

•**Confirmation of the actual duration of pregnancy.** Measurement of the fetal crown-rump length during the first three months of pregnancy gives, with an accuracy of plus or minus four days, the date of conception! After the first three months, measurement of the head size (biparietal diameter), the abdominal circumference, and the length of a femur (long leg bone) will reveal the same information. In later pregnancy, two ultrasound examinations six weeks apart can also provide a very accurate assessment of fetal age except in cases of IUGR (discussed later in this section). Knowing the true duration of pregnancy is of great importance in risk situations in which an early delivery is indicated. Further, accurate dating determines once and for all when pregnancy is *truly* going overdue. This knowledge has significant clinical as well as social importance.

A head-on look at an umbilical cord cross section. The arrows direct us to three black circles representing the three blood vessels (two arteries and a vein) that are always present in a normal cord.

•**Estimating the fetal weight.** Using a variety of measurements, fetal weight can be estimated to within a few ounces of actual weight.

•**Determination of intrauterine growth retardation (IUGR).** This condition may develop in a number of abnormal obstetrical circumstances, usually after the 28th week. It may be due to fetal damage from many sources in early pregnancy or to failure of placental function in later pregnancy from a number of disorders. IUGR, a very important obstetrical complication, is discussed further on pages 160–161.

•**Identification of multiple pregnancies.** Twins, triplets, and more are identified almost absolutely by ultrasound. Note, though, that "twins" are sometimes seen on early ultrasound examination, only to have one of them disappear a little later because one represents a false fetal sac. This is very new information. It is possible that many pregnancies start out *appearing* as twins. So when an early ultrasound picture suggests twins, it needs to be repeated later.

•**Investigation of abnormal bleeding.** In late pregnancy and even in early pregnancy, ultrasound is used to locate the area of placental implantation or to locate other sources of abnormal bleeding.

•**Location of IUDs.** Ultrasound is used to identify, locate, and document the presence and location of an intrauterine contraceptive device (IUD), which can sometimes complicate a pregnancy.

•**Establishing fetal age and well-being.** Prior to attempting certain surgical procedures to close the cervix (cerclage) in some types of recurrent premature labor, the fetal well-being and age need to be clearly established.

•**Tumors and cysts.** Ultrasound is used to determine the potential for causing harm and the nature of certain pelvic tumors and cysts of the reproductive organs. Ultrasound examination can assist in defining the characteristics of these growths and their potential for interfering with pregnancy.

•**Identifying fetal abnormalities and disorders.** Gross abnormalities and, nowadays, even small structural defects are being delineated by ultrasound.

•**Determining the biophysical profile (BPP).** Advanced ultrasound analysis of fetal activity is now available in most obstetrical services throughout our country. Such analysis, carried out by skilled sonographers, measures many variables in the intrauterine environment and is reported in scores of 1–10 as a biophysical profile (BPP). Included are many fetal measurements, amniotic fluid volume, placental age, fetal breathing, and movement activity such as hand grasping, and more. The result of all this data is a very useful assessment of fetal well-being. Its use is generally reserved for the last trimester of high-risk pregnancies. It may well be that the BPP will replace stress and nonstress testing in the future.

•**The potential for premature labor.** Transvaginal ultrasound of the cervix in the late second trimester provides valuable information concerning the likelihood of premature labor. This is of value in managing plural pregnancies and women with a history of cervical incompetence (see page 233). The cervical length can be accurately measured at this examination and the length helps predict the risk of premature labor—the shorter it is, the more likely is early labor.

•**Transabdominal procedures.** Amniocentesis, CVS, all manner of rapidly developing intrauterine fetal surgery, placental studies—all these procedures and more would be impossible without ultrasound guidance.

•**Determination of sex.** The high resolution obtained in modern ultrasound can determine, with accuracy, the sex of the fetus. This is usually confined to last-trimester ultrasound procedures and is not considered an important diagnostic yield—except, perhaps, in certain sex-linked disorders.

•**Confirmation of fetal position.** Sometimes it becomes important to know the exact position in which the fetus lies. As an example, "external cephalic version" is a procedure sometimes undertaken in order to manually turn a breech (bottom) to a vertex (head) presentation by abdominal manipulations. This turning—when successful—can make a difficult labor much simpler. The procedure must be done before labor, with the breech not engaged in the pelvis, and the operator who is about to do the abdominal turning or version must know exactly how the baby lies and exactly where the placenta lies.

•**Placental health and location.** Knowledge of the placental location is important in many ways. Transabdominal procedures must avoid the placenta, and as indicated in the previous paragraph, abdominal manipulations require knowledge of its exact position. The precise location is also important if there is any abnormal vaginal bleeding in order to rule out a placenta previa. Placental aging and circulation can be determined by ultrasound; this becomes important in IUGR, post-term, and other problematic pregnancies. It has also become significant to determine the umbilical cord's point of insertion into the placenta. Insertions that are extremely lateral or even on the membranes themselves (velamentous) can adversely affect the pregnancy. Finally, the degree of umbilical cord coiling is regarded as an indication of fetal health. The more coiling, the better. Very interestingly, European obstetricians have been able to surgically separate twin placentas within the uterus. This has been done when evidence revealed that one twin was regularly stealing from the other twin's placenta! Now, that is amazing.

Doppler Ultrasound

Doppler ultrasound is another method of evaluating fetal health. This technique, the result of our advancing technology, sends sound waves that strike red blood cells as they move about in the maternal and fetal circulation. Arterial blood flows faster than venous blood, and this provides a different image for each. Computers translate this flow-rate differential into color, and so we see arterial blood as red and venous blood as blue. Thus, we can study uterine and umbilical circulation. Calculation of the red cell flow-rates yields very basic information about many abnormal obstetrical states. IUGR, hypertension of pregnancy, and fetal heart anomalies are just some of the conditions being studied by this new and very helpful technique. Doppler procedures have been found to be useful in studying circulatory problems in all parts of our own bodies.

Routine Pregnancy Ultrasound or Not?

Ultrasound observations in pregnancy proliferated rapidly after reasonably good machines became available at reasonable prices. Today they are found in most obstetricians' offices, all radiology clinics, and all obstetrical units. A good office ultrasound costs at least $35,000, but a state-of-the-art machine can cost $250,000 and is not found in doctors' offices!

The ultrasound cost to the patient varies widely but on average runs about $200—sometimes borne by insurance or HMOs, sometimes not.

Early on it was argued that a routine ultrasound in every pregnancy was neither cost-effective nor revealing. Sonograms for every pregnancy would cost over $1 billion each year, and, of further importance, several studies failed to document worthwhile information coming from this approach. With more recent studies, however, that position has somewhat changed. Better equipment and better skills have apparently confirmed the value of this procedure in detecting fetal anomalies and unsuspected plural pregnancies. These and other developing long-term benefits are apparently approaching cost-effectiveness.

Ultrasound Safety

At the beginning of this section, we said that ultrasound is a safe procedure. And so it is. Ultrasound is energy. Such energy delivered to a fetus varies with the sound frequency, intensity, duration of exposure, and distance from the source (the transducer). Such exposures, using standard present-day equipment, have not been found to cause any harmful biological effects on pregnant women, their fetuses, or the sonographers who repeatedly do these procedures. The infants exposed during pregnancy have shown no differences in any measurable way from unexposed infants after decades of follow-up.

It must be pointed out, however, that newer applications and instruments are requiring higher outputs of energy, higher enough that these machines now continuously display the level of energy they are producing and the operators are advised to use as little energy as is prudent—whatever prudent may be! Again, at this time there have been no reports of any fetal, maternal, or operator damage from these powerful new devices.

Fetal Monitoring

Physicians have always been vitally interested in intrauterine fetal activity—in particular, the beating fetal heart. In the past we used stethoscopes to listen for fetal activity and fetal heartbeat. Before that our listening devices were rolled-up pieces of stout paper, such as you now find lining shirts back fresh from the laundry (if your laundry still provides that nice little touch). By putting one end to the ear and the other on the mother's abdomen, the doctor could hear an abundance of fetal activity.

Some casual or more daring physicians in the past directly applied their ear to the mother's abdomen, and it would yield the same information—even more clearly. Today, however, most external monitoring is done with ultrasound devices that bounce echoes off the fetal heart valves; the echoes are translated into an audible beat that can be clearly heard by both mother and physician—a very delightful sensation indeed.

The fetal heart begins to beat at about the sixth week of pregnancy and can be heard as early as the tenth week with standard equipment. It can be heard much earlier with more sophisticated devices, depending on some variable factors that have nothing to do with the well-being of the fetus—such as the thickness of the mother's abdomen and the position of the uterus. Nevertheless, it is the standard devices that are used at each visit to listen for the fetal heart rate and sometimes for certain other things, such as the placenta location.

As pregnancy progresses, the heart rate becomes of more and more critical interest and value. There are many things going on inside that affect the maternal-fetal environment and are reflected by the fetal heart rate and variability. This is particularly true in infants being stressed by an internal environment that does not deliver enough food, oxygen, or both and, further, does not remove waste metabolic products on a regular basis.

Although great placental reserves are present to protect the fetus, certain conditions, such as chronic malnutrition, diabetes, high blood pressure, chronic alcohol, drug, or tobacco poisoning, and, as we shall see, many other problems, can obliterate such placental reserves as time and injury go on. Signs of reserve depletion usually appear after the 28th week, and the development of techniques to monitor and interpret heart rate values beyond this point has become a science unto itself.

There are a number of tests for placental reserve and function.

Nonstress Test (NST)

First of all, some definitions: *fetal stress* means that something is going on in the fetal environment that is stressing the fetus in some way. The stress could be caused by an aging placenta, maternal illness such as diabetes or starvation, social poisonings (alcohol or tobacco, for example), or any number of things. The infant reacts to such stress in several ways, one of which is reflected in its heart rate.

Stress is not necessarily damaging, any more than stress is to adults—up to a certain point. Repeated and continued stress, however, can lead to *fetal distress*. In this situation, the stress has continued and/or increased to a point where the fetus is in some real jeopardy and intervention may be required.

A nonstress test attempts to measure fetal well-being without adding to any other stress that may already be affecting the fetus. This procedure can be done in the labor suite or in your doctor's office. An external ultrasound monitor is placed over the abdomen in the fetal heart area, and heartbeats are recorded on a monitoring strip of paper. This paper recording is the only thing that differs from the regular heart monitor that the doctor has previously used to listen to your baby.

It is now known that, under normal circumstances, fetal heart activity waxes and wanes with periods of wakefulness and sleep as well as during fetal movement. These episodes occur at more or less regular intervals. In a healthy pregnancy, then, the heart rate increases during periods of fetal activity and will appear on the monitoring strip. When this normal reaction is observed, we have a *reactive NST.* It indicates that the fetus is at present under no stress. On the other hand, failure of the heartbeat to speed up indicates a potential fetal problem and is designated a *nonreactive NST.*

Such tests are repeated every few days or weekly, depending on the circumstances and indications, but if they become nonreactive, we move on.

Contraction Stress Test (CST)

The CST is based upon the response of the fetal heart rate to uterine contractions. This procedure actually puts a certain amount of stress on the placenta, and therefore the baby, and by so doing determines whether fetal distress is present or imminent. This is the procedure to be followed if the NST becomes nonreactive, and its purpose is to indicate the possibility that placental reserve is significantly diminished and the fetal environment is compromised.

In order to produce stress, the uterus is made to contract, much as it would in labor. To do this, we must start an intravenous infusion and administer oxytocin, the drug used to accelerate or induce labor. Further, we add to the monitoring devices a gauge to determine the duration and amplitude of our induced uterine contractions. Under healthy circumstances, the fetal heart rate does not decline with a normal and customary uterine contraction. If, however, it is being deprived and therefore distressed during a contraction, the heartbeat drops and we have a positive oxytocin challenge test (OCT) or contraction stress test (CST). (Either designation, OCT or CST, means the same thing.) Any positive challenge test becomes a signal for an immediate full-scale review of the pregnancy.

Breast Stimulation Test (BST)

It is known that nipple stimulation produces uterine contractions by making the natural oxytocin substance appear in maternal blood; that's why afterpains are sharper while you nurse. We can therefore achieve the same results as the standard challenge test but without having to start an intravenous and without running the slight risk of excessive uterine contractions from the oxytocin medication. This simplified breast stimulation test is easier to perform and can be an office procedure. The mother is asked to gently stimulate one nipple (through her clothing) for a two-minute period. This is generally sufficient to produce a contraction and so no intravenous hookup is necessary. This much simpler procedure can be accomplished in half the time it takes to do a CST, and at considerably less expense.

Acoustic Fetal Stimulation

This is a relatively new irritant technique that further invades and disturbs the tranquillity of the fetal environment to see how things are going. A variety of measured noise-producing devices are beamed to the fetus through the maternal abdomen. Just as an alarm clock would affect us, the fetus is similarly disturbed by this auditory insult. Its response is measured by the cardiac and motion activity that follow this clarion call. Although there has been some question about auditory damage—even terror—to the fetus, no adverse statistics have been established and the procedure seems to be gathering advocates.

Biophysical Profile (BPP)

The BPP is a very thorough assessment of fetal well-being. It usually has five components:

1. A nonstress test (NST)

2. Observations of regular fetal breathing

3. Observations of fetal movements

4. Fetal tone—extension and flexion of extremities

5. Amniotic fluid volume and placental grading

These five areas of study—usually requiring 30 minutes minimum—are each graded 0–2. Thus, 10 is a perfect score; 8–10 is normal; 6–8 is

At right is a typical sonographer's report form that is completed for a Biophysical Profile (BPP). The report is signed by the ultrasound technician and by the radiologist responsible for the data accumulation and the final score. In this particular report, six items are evaluated and a perfect BPP would be 12. Some institutions report the Nonstress Test (NST) separately; the perfect BPP would then be 10. Qualitative AFI is a measurement of the amniotic fluid volume.

OB Ultrasound Exam

Patient Name: _____ G ____ P ____ A ____
LMP: _____ Exam Date: _____
MR: _____ Referring MD: _____

General Evaluation

Fetal Cardiac Activity: _____ BPM
Placental Location: _____ Grade: _____
Amniotic Fluid Volume: _____ cm: _____
Fetal Presentation: _____
Cervical Length: _____

Biometry

BPD: _____ mm	Gest. Age: _____ wks	HC/AC: _____
HC: _____ mm	Gest. Age: _____ wks	FL/BPD: _____
AC: _____ mm	Gest. Age: _____ wks	FL/AC: _____
FL: _____ mm	Gest. Age: _____ wks	
CRL: _____ mm	Gest. Age: _____ wks	
SAC: _____ mm	Gest. Age: _____ wks	
Yolk sac: _____	Adnexa: _____	

Clinical EDC: _____ Gest. Age: _____ wks _____ days _____
Composite ultrasound EDC: _____ Gest. Age: _____ wks _____ days _____

Fetal Weight: ____ grams (+/- grams) FFW: _____ % based on clinical EDC

Fetal Anatomy

Cranium: _____	Bladder: _____
Ventricles: _____	Abd Cord Ins: _____
Cerebellum: _____	Cord Vessels: _____
Spine: _____	Kidneys: _____
Heart: _____	Orbits: _____
Stomach: _____	Extremities: _____

Biophysical Profile

(Normal–2, Abnormal=0)

Fetal Tone: _____
Gross Body Movements: _____
Fetal Breathing Movements: _____
Qualitative AFI: _____
Nonstress Test: _____
TOTAL SCORE: _____

Comments: _____

_____
_____
_____
_____

Technologist: _____ MD: _____

marginal, and the test needs to be repeated within 24 hours; 5 or less is abnormal and active intervention is required.

A less cumbersome, modified BPP is based on the following observation: In the third trimester, amniotic fluid reflects fetal urine production. Decreased placental function decreases fetal renal clearance and therefore decreases urine output. The end result is oligohydramnios (diminished amniotic fluid). Therefore, the modified BPP involves only a NST and a measurement of amniotic fluid levels.

Ante-partum fetal monitoring is of value and finds use in many situations, some of which were mentioned earlier. Here is a more complete list of its indications:

- decreased fetal movements

- maternal hypertensive disorders

- diabetes

- oligohydramnios

- IUGR (intrauterine growth retardation)

- postmature pregnancies (over 42 weeks)

- maternal renal disease

- certain isoimmunization problems—Rh factor, for instance

- significant maternal heart disease

- pleural pregnancies with discordant fetal growth patterns

- certain other maternal systemic disorders such as hyperthyroidism and lupus erythematosis

- previous unexplained fetal loss

The selection, timing, and frequency of any of these fetal tests depends on many circumstances that only your personal obstetrician can assess.

(Some of the material in this section was derived from the American College of Obstetricians and Gynecologists' *Technical Bulletin*, no. 188, 1994.)

Fetal Monitoring in Labor

In normal as well as abnormal labor, the monitoring equipment just described above for CSTs is used almost routinely to observe fetal heart rate and maternal uterine contraction activity. Fetal monitoring is a relatively reliable indicator of the infant's well-being during labor and delivery and also provides a record of maternal uterine activity while labor is progressing. The fetal heart rate pattern shows accelerations and decelerations under a variety of labor conditions, and these recorded observations are of certain value in protecting and guarding fetal well-being during the critical labor and delivery period.

Many arguments are being raised today about routine fetal monitoring during labor. It has been declared that such monitoring has shown no significant fetal benefits and has contributed to the increased rate of cesarean section. It has certainly increased the rate of litigation as doctors, lawyers, judges, and juries attempt to resolve the argument. A fairly recent position paper issued by the American College of Obstetricians and Gynecologists concludes that electronic fetal monitoring offers no significant advantages in normal labor over that provided by regular listening with a stethoscope. It may be that various investigators and clinicians have attempted to read too much into fetal cardiac patterns as labor progresses. Moreover, many have coined their own terms to describe various fetal heart patterns—much like an artist describing colors.

At any rate, in order to untangle this web we have spun, the National Institutes of Health (NIH) appointed a committee of experts to sort all these things out and to provide a set of principles that will:

- assure the reliability of monitoring when tracings are read by different people

- confirm the validity of monitoring in associated specific heart rate patterns with adverse neurological outcomes

- determine whether interventions based on monitor tracings will help avoid adverse fetal outcomes

This committee has worked diligently for the past three years and will publish its findings and recommendations sometime in 1998. In the meantime, fetal and contraction monitoring will likely continue and increase.

Home Uterine Activity Monitoring (HUAM)

Premature labor and, thus, prematurity are such a major obstetrical problem that we look for help from any potential procedure in order to prevent it. One of these procedures is HUAM—home uterine monitoring.

When premature labor is anticipated, such as with plural pregnancies, a weakened, incompetent cervix, or a history of premature labor, HUAM has been advocated as a safeguard procedure that identifies threatening contractions in time for tocolytic (contraction-stopping) hospital treatments. A device strapped to the maternal abdomen records uterine contraction activity and each day the wearer calls in the data collected to the doctor's office. These data are scanned by competent observers and decisions made upon the findings.

Over a dozen studies have failed to provide us with a firm answer as to the worth of this monitoring procedure, but the weight of evidence seems to be gradually shifting in its favor. It is certainly a painless and safe program, and I hope it will continue to flourish as more evidence about its worth is accumulated.

Fetoscopy and Fetal Surgery

With the advent of all the new techniques of evaluating fetal health and activity within the uterus, it became a challenge to see whether we could extend our diagnostic arm even further and perhaps extend a therapeutic arm along with it. The result is a brand-new specialty—fetology. This specialty, as the term indicates, is the study of unborn babies. There are few fetologists in this country, and very few centers where fetology and its operative extensions, fetoscopy and fetal surgery, can be undertaken. *Fetoscopy* is a technique whereby the uterus is entered and the fetus observed directly with a fiber-optic lighted lens and a grasping apparatus, often equipped with the capability of taking certain samples—even performing some surgery. In reality, it is a modified operative laparoscope. The fetoscope is inserted through the mother's abdomen and uterus. This direct visualization allows for the certain detection of many types of structural defects. The samples that may be obtained consist of:

- blood taken from the placental vessels, which is used to help determine certain types of blood disorders, such as sickle cell anemia, thalassemia, and destructive blood disorders

- skin biopsies, removed to evaluate genetic skin disorders and used in genetic analysis

- muscle biopsies, taken to detect some forms of cerebral palsy

- liver biopsies, analyzed for certain metabolic disorders

Fetoscopy Risks

The maternal risks are slight, believe it or not. Infection may occur, but this is unusual. Fetal risk consists of a 5 percent chance that premature labor and, as a consequence, fetal demise may follow. These risks must be weighed carefully against the derived benefits.

Fetal Surgery

For the past decade or so, fetal surgery has been performed by some fetologists. These techniques have been developed in order to try to save some unborn infants with problems that might otherwise make their survival out of the uterus impossible. Examples include:

- **Hydrocephalus management.** The head is so distended with fluid that a safe delivery, by any route, is virtually impossible. Fetologists can drain the fluid away and, after a safe delivery, manage the disorder permanently.

- **Congenital bladder obstructions** can lead to urinary backup and kidney destruction. This can be overcome by placing stents or tubes into the bladder and then doing corrective surgery after delivery.

- Laser surgery occludes **abnormal placental blood vessels** and separates twin placentas when one is parasiting the other.

- When an infant is in jeopardy from **destructive genetic blood disorders,** laser surgery allows stem-cell transfusions.

- It also allows whole blood transfusions in certain **Rh situations.**

New procedures are being added all the time; this is just a representative list of what can be done in this amazing field of endeavor. As always, the risks and benefits must be carefully weighed when these procedures are contemplated, and the mother and father must be willing, informed participants in any decision-making process.

The delicate work of fetoscopy and fetoscopic surgery demands special institutions and qualified fetologists. Therefore, go only to a tertiary care facility (see discussion later in the appendix)—one equipped with all the technical expertise and equipment that fetoscopy involves—and work only with skilled fetologists with superb ultrasound techniques as well as good clinical skills in using labor-inhibiting drugs, so as to prevent uterine contractions and premature expulsion of the infant under study.

Progress in fetology and fetal surgery in America is slow, as a variety of risks and rewards are being reevaluated. In Europe, however, fetologists are rapidly forging ahead with procedures once considered impossible.

The Blood Shed (Cord Blood Storage)

"Stem" cells in the body's blood-generation programs are the progenitor cells that have multi-potential capabilities to make new blood cells. They are found in human bone marrow, where our new blood is normally built. They are also found in profusion in human fetal umbilical cord blood. These cord stem cells have several advantages, for treatment purposes, over bone marrow. They are less likely to carry adult diseases, and they are less immunogenic—that is, less likely to cause a host/graft rejection disorder. Compared again to bone marrow, they are certainly much more easily and painlessly obtainable, being thrown away by the barrel each day. Since it became clear that cord blood could be used instead of bone marrow for transplant procedures, it became worthwhile to consider storage of this blood. Accordingly, "blood sheds" were made available for frozen storage both as a research vehicle and as a private source of cord blood in case a child needs it later for treatment of a blood disease or in case a family member needs stem cell replacement for any number of medical problems, including cancer and cancer treatment. Thus, cord blood may now be privately stored at a cost of $1,500 initially and $100 per year thereafter. Those costs will surely change as time goes by. The cord blood is taken after delivery of the placenta by a sterile technique that deposits the blood into a sterile container, then sends it off to be properly tested identified, frozen, and stored.

This new program has raised many medical, ethical, and financial problems. Here are a few:

- There is a very low probability that the infant donor will ever need the blood.

- Will the frozen blood be good in 18–25 years?

- Will the cord specimen have enough blood to fulfill adult needs?

- The low host/graft resistance also represents a less-active immune capability of the cord cells. Will this make it less useful in transplants to adult cancer victims?

- A good number of cord blood specimens are contaminated with maternal blood at collection. What effect will this have on future graft acceptance?

- Can cord blood be collected for commercial use in the future without consent?

And so it goes. A great deal of this story has yet to unfold, and it will be interesting to see what new information and developments may be described in the sixth edition! Clearly, some of the questions about cord blood storage will soon be answered—and easily so. Others will be difficult to answer, if indeed they are ever answered before cancer treatment moves beyond bridgeheads such as this cold cord storage provides. For the present, it appears to be an exciting concept.

Perinatal (Tertiary Care) Centers

In order to deliver maternal health care in the most effective way possible, and at the least possible cost, doctors have instituted a nationwide network of perinatal centers. At the hub of each center is a class III maternity unit. These tertiary care centers, as they are also known, can manage the most critical obstetrical problems. The staff is skilled in maternal-fetal medicine (perinatology), special infant care (neonatology), and obstetrical anesthesia. Further, all laboratory and support equipment this type of service may require, such as level II ultrasound, is readily available.

In the communities surrounding each tertiary care center, there are many secondary and primary obstetrical hospitals. A primary care hospital (class I) usually manages normal obstetrical patients. Secondary hospitals (class II), on the other hand, are involved in the management of some complicated obstetrical problems, and their doctors perform operative procedures. Serious and dangerous complications, however, are referred up the chain to the tertiary care center. Thus, doctors practicing even in very remote areas of our country know that there is a big brother always ready and available to assist them and their mothers with major problems. Ambulances, helicopters, and computer networks are an integral part of each network.

As an example, the University of Tennessee Medical Center in Memphis is the tertiary care center for western Tennessee, eastern Arkansas, and northern Mississippi. If you look at a regional map, you will see why this location makes geographic sense. Almost every corner of the United States is thus organized to ensure the very best obstetrical care in the world to American mothers.

If this is so, you may wonder why it is that the United States still rates 22nd—second to last—in the world in fetal mortality figures. The answer to that is not to be found in the health care delivery system. It lies in our lifestyle, our dietary and social habits, our diverse racial population, and our enormous adolescent pregnancy population. Moreover, no other country reports its fetal mortality as faithfully and as fully as we do.

Glossary

The glossary defines many of the terms used throughout this book. Italicized words within a definition are defined elsewhere in the glossary.

ABORTION Loss of a pregnancy, either accidentally or purposefully, before viability (20 weeks).

ACIDOSIS A state of metabolic imbalance that may occur in diabetics, during prolonged labor, or in the *fetus* under certain circumstances, such as placental insufficiency or other causes of oxygen deprivation.

AFP See *Alpha Fetoprotein*.

AFTERBIRTH See *Placenta*.

ALBUMINURIA Albumen (a protein) in the urine—an abnormal finding often associated with kidney disorders and with *toxemia* (*preeclampsia*) of pregnancy.

ALPHA-FETOPROTEIN (AFP) A substance secreted by the *fetus* that becomes enclosed in its spinal canal system during early body development. Its presence in the maternal blood and in the amniotic fluid should diminish and disappear after the spinal canal normally closes. Its presence is used, then, to indicate the health of the fetal spinal canal and cranial system.

AMNIOCENTESIS Needle aspiration of *amniotic fluid* through the mother's abdomen for *chromosome* culture and many other tests.

AMNIOTIC FLUID Liquid surrounding the *fetus,* composed of secretions from the *placenta*, fetal urine and other minor constituents.

ANALGESIA Relief of pain without loss of consciousness.

ANESTHESIA Complete relief of pain by either general or local agents; complete loss of consciousness under general anesthesia.

ANTIBODIES Protein warriors formed by the body to defend against similar protein invaders—the basic principle of vaccination. May go astray in the Rh incompatibility problems.

APGAR SCORE A method of rating a baby's condition at birth and five or more minutes later. It is the summation of a number of observed factors in the newborn, such as heart rate, respiratory rate, color, muscle activity, and so on. A perfect score would be 10–10—rarely achieved.

AREOLA. Pigmented skin area around breast nipples, which darkens during pregnancy. Montgomery follicles may appear in the areola. These are little raised white areas of no consequence.

AUTOSOMES Another name for *chromosomes,* excluding the sex chromosomes.

BABY BLUES See *depression.*

BARR BODY Females have two X *chromosomes,* but usually only one works. The other, which curls into a ball in the bottom of each cell's nucleus, is called a Barr body.

BETA HCG A highly specific fragment of the *human chorionic gonadotropin* (HCG) complex that is very important in assessing (1) the presence of pregnancy, (2) the health of the fetus, (3) the diagnosis of an ectopic pregnancy, and (4) along with other blood tests, the presence of Down's syndrome.

BILIRUBIN Everybody has some bilirubin in their blood, but an excess hemoglobin breakdown in newborns may produce excess bilirubin and jaundice—even without Rh disorders. The excess is generally treated by exposure to light, rarely by exchange transfusion.

BIOPHYSICAL PROFILE (BPP) A significant test for fetal well-being done in an *ultrasound* laboratory. Five different fetal conditions and activities are measured to achieve the final score. The test is usually done after the 28th week and is often repeated as term approaches. Also called fetal biophysical profile (FBP).

BONDING The psychological union of the mother, father, and child at the time of birth when they first all touch, see, hear, and feel one another. It is most desirable to bond immediately after birth, but there are some excellent alternatives if this cannot be done.

BRAXTON-HICKS CONTRACTIONS Usually painless, sometimes painful, usually irregular, sometimes regular *contractions* of the *uterus.* They begin early in pregnancy and continue throughout, helping to force blood through the uterus.

BREAST STIMULATION TEST A relatively safe, noninvasive method of determining fetal well-being in the last trimester. Self-stimulation of the mother's nipple produces uterine *contractions,* and concurrent monitoring of the fetal heart rate indicates the baby's reaction to the stress of such a contraction.

BREECH A not uncommon presentation of a baby, in which the bottom instead of the head comes forth first.

CANDIDA ALBICANS Commonest cause of yeast infections in the vagina—likely to occur in pregnancy.

CATHETER A plastic or rubber tube to draw urine from the bladder. May be left in place (in-dwelling) postpartum for a day or so if an operative delivery is necessary.

CAUDAL A form of *epidural anesthetic* administered very low in the epidural space.

CAUTERIZATION Electro-coagulation of infected tissue—usually cervical tissue—to produce healing.

CEPHALO-PELVIC DISPROPORTION (CPD) The condition when the presenting part or parts of the baby do not satisfactorily fit into the maternal pelvic bone and tissue structures.

CERVICAL OS The muscular fibrous ring of the cervix that keeps the *uterus* closed until *labor* begins.

CERVIX Neck of the womb (*uterus*)—the uterine opening into the upper vagina.

CESAREAN SECTION A surgical delivery through an abdominal incision rather than the normal vaginal route.

CHLOASMA Darkening of areas of the skin during pregnancy—usually the breast areola, forehead, cheeks, and abdomen.

CHORIONIC SAMPLING A modern method of determining the genetic makeup of an *embryo*. Through the *cervix*, by a variety of techniques, direct samples are taken of the chorion—the fetal tissue that will form the *placenta*. This procedure can be done very early in pregnancy (at ten weeks). The samples are then analyzed genetically to determine the presence, or absence, of inherited disorders.

CHROMOSOME Each cell has 23 pairs of chromosomes. They carry the *genes*, which carry all the inherited characteristics.

CLASTOGEN A drug or substance that can damage a *fetus* without necessarily producing a visible defect.

COLOSTRUM The forerunner of milk, present in the breast as early as the second month.

CONCEPTION The union of a ripe ovum with a sperm to form a new life.

CONDYLOMATA ACUMINATA A viral infection (the human papilloma virus) that produces warts at the entrance of the vagina and sometimes in the vagina itself.

CONTRACTION STRESS TEST (CST) See *Fetal Stress Test* (FST).

CONTRACTION (UTERINE) The *uterus* contracts throughout most of pregnancy, generally nonpainless *Braxton-Hicks contractions*. Sometimes such contractions are regular and produce false labor, but when true labor begins, the contractions become closer and harder as uterine evacuation begins.

CORD BLOOD STORAGE An innovative program involving the collection of umbilical and placental blood after delivery, then freezing and storing it for future use in place of bone marrow in the management of various cancers. Although this program is set up and running, there is still a great deal to be learned about it.

CORPUS LUTEUM CYST A normal ovarian cyst that forms each month on the ovary at the point where ovulation occurs. It grows for the first three months of pregnancy, supporting the pregnancy, then disappears. It may cause some pain in early pregnancy.

COUVADE SYNDROME The sharing of the symptoms of early pregnancy by the father.

CPD See *Cephalo-Pelvic Disproportion.*

CYTOMEGALOVIRUS This sexually transmitted virus can cause certain problems related to infertility and to specific birth defects.

DELIVERY The act of expulsion of the baby, either through the vagina or through a *cesarean section* incision.

DEPRESSION A feeling of helplessness and hopelessness that can come over anyone at any time. It may occur during early pregnancy and soon after delivery but is usually temporary unless there is an undercurrent of previous depression. Whatever the degree of symptoms, it must not be neglected.

DIAPHRAGM A fairly effective birth control device.

DIAPHRAGMATIC HERNIA A hiatus or epigastric hernia. Stomach tissue is pushed into the chest through the muscular diaphragm, which separates the chest from the abdomen. It often occurs temporarily in late pregnancy.

DILATION The degree of openness of the *cervix.* Usually closed until labor begins, the cervix dilates from one to ten centimeters during labor.

DIURETIC A medication that removes water from the body—usually not indicated in pregnancy except under certain special conditions.

DIZYGOTIC TWINS Fraternal twins—two babies from two separate eggs.

DOWN'S SYNDROME (MONGOLISM) A genetic birth defect, sometimes sporadic, sometimes inherited, much more common in babies of mothers over 35. It is due to a translocation (abnormal location) of certain genes.

ECTOPIC PREGNANCY A pregnancy that implants anywhere outside the uterus—most commonly in a fallopian tube but also possible in an ovary or even in the abdomen.

EDC See *Expected Date of Confinement.*

EDEMA Swelling of body tissues due to the retention of fluid.

ELECTROLYTES Dissolved salts, buffering acids, or alkalis normally found in the blood plasma or tissue fluids.

EMBRYO A living human being that results from *conception* and, if it remains in place, leads to one of us.

EPIDURAL ANESTHETIC Unlike a spinal block, an epidural doesn't enter the spinal canal but blocks nerve impulses as they leave it. It has few side effects and usually offers the best type of pain relief for labor. A *caudal* is a particular form of epidural anesthetic.

EPIGASTRIC HERNIA See *diaphragmatic hernia.*

EPISIOTOMY An incision made in the *perineum* to prevent tears in that area or in the rectum and surrounding tissues during labor.

EXPECTED DATE OF CONFINEMENT (EDC) or EXPECTED DATE OF DELIVERY (EDD) Give or take a week or two.

FALLOPIAN TUBES The tubes that conduct eggs to the *uterus.* Fertilization usually occurs in the tubes—and most ectopics come to rest there.

FETAL BIOPHYSICAL PROFILE (FBP) See *Biophysical Profile* (BPP).

FETAL MONITORS Electronic devices that, when attached by proper leads and sensing devices on the mother's abdominal wall, measure uterine *contractions* and fetal heart rate during labor. At some point in *labor,* when the *cervix* is sufficiently dilated, the fetal sensor may be applied directly to the fetal scalp. Moreover, sometimes direct internal measurement of uterine contraction activity is possible by placing a very soft sensor high into the uterus—again, through the opened cervix. Most labors in the United States are monitored. Fetal electronic monitors are also an integral part of the fetal stress test (FST), as well as the nonstress test (NST).

FETAL STRESS TEST (FST) A procedure to determine the presence of fetal stress or distress in late pregnancy. Using intravenous pitocin, an oxytocin, uterine *contractions* are produced and the fetal heart rate response to the contractions is measured and interpreted. This particular test is also known as a contraction stress test (CST) or an oxytocin challenge test (OCT).

FETOLOGY The study of unborn infants in their intrauterine environment.

FETOSCOPY A relatively new science that studies the *fetus* and its uterine environment with a variety of invasive instruments. May be compared to laparoscopy or arthroscopy in principle.

FETUS An unborn child.

FORCEPS Safe (in skilled hands) tong-like instruments used to extract babies late in labor. Occasionally—and more rarely nowadays—used to turn babies lying in abnormal positions.

FST See *Fetal Stress Test.*

GENES Ultra structures made up of DNA, which are present on *chromosome* strands and control inherited characteristics.

GERMAN MEASLES (RUBELLA) A simple viral disease that is of little significance unless it occurs during pregnancy. In early pregnancy in particular it can cause marked birth defects.

GRAVIDA The number of times a patient has been pregnant. For example, "gravida 10" means ten conceptions, regardless of the outcome.

HCG See *Human Chorionic Gonadotropin.*

HERPES VIRUS II A highly communicable venereal disease for which there is still no cure. The obstetrical risk is significant when this disease is active. Should there be an open herpes ulcer on the cervix, in the vagina, or on the vaginal entrance at the time of delivery, a *cesarean section* should be performed to safeguard the child from the possibility of developing systemic herpes after it passes through the birth canal.

HIATUS HERNIA See *diaphragmatic hernia.*

HUMAN CHORIONIC GONADOTROPIN The hormone of pregnancy secreted by the *placenta,* which produces the first positive evidence of pregnancy.

HYALINE MEMBRANE DISEASE Coating of fetal lungs that prevents adequate oxygen exchange. More common in premature infants, after *cesarean section,* and in some other obstetrical conditions. Also called respiratory distress syndrome (RDS).

HYDRAMNIOS Excess amounts of *amniotic fluid* surrounding the baby; it may mean nothing, or it may signify fetal defects.

HYPERTENSION Elevation of resting blood pressure levels above normal limits—high blood pressure.

HYPERTENSION OF PREGNANCY Often known as *toxemia* or *preeclampsia* and eclampsia, this condition, peculiar to human pregnancy, is characterized *by hypertension, edema,* and protein in the urine—all usually developing in the last trimester.

INDUCTION OF LABOR The artificial initiation of labor for any reason.

INTRAUTERINE DEVICE (IUD) A plastic, metallic/plastic, or hormonal device inserted into the *uterus* for birth control.

LABOR Productive uterine contractions that normally cause dilation of the *cervix,* descent of the baby, and its expulsion into the world.

LA LECHE LEAGUE A national group of individuals devoted to the encouragement of breast-feeding.

LAMAZE METHOD An obstetrical learning program which prepares mothers and their partners for the labor experience.

LANUGO Downy soft hair that coats the fetal body.

LEBOYER METHOD A quiet, peaceful delivery experience designed to reduce birth trauma to infants.

LECITHIN A substance present in high ratios when fetal lungs arc mature.

LIGHTENING When the baby drops into the pelvis and the mother can breathe again. Usually taking place in the last month of pregnancy, it may happen suddenly (in a few hours) or over a period of days.

LOCHIA Vaginal secretions of blood and fluids that persist after delivery on and off until the first menstrual flow. Never heavier than a menstrual flow or excessively irritating.

MISCARRIAGE An accidental abortion.

MONGOLISM See *Down's Syndrome.*

MONOZYGOTIC TWINS Identical twins, coming from one ovum or egg.

MORNING SICKNESS Half of all mothers have it moderately, and a few severely, during the first few months. Consisting of nausea and/or vomiting, it is usually most bothersome in the early morning but sometimes lasts all day.

MYCOPLASMOSIS A rare vaginal infection that can interfere with fertility and reproduction.

NEONATOLOGIST A pediatric specialist who is especially trained to take care of distressed newborn babies.

NONSTRESS TEST (NST) At present, the most commonly used technique to assess fetal well-being during late pregnancy. A *fetus* with a normal central nervous system, unblunted by oxygen deprivation or acidosis, moves about regularly within the *uterus.* Such movements are accompanied by accelerations of the fetal heart rate, and, of course, the changing heart rate appears on a fetal monitoring device. Measurement of these basal heart rate changes therefore indicates the presence or absence of fetal distress. It is called a nonstress test because no uterine contractions are induced in an NST—such as are done in a *fetal stress test* (FST).

OBSTETRICIAN A medical doctor who specializes in the management of pregnancy and childbirth. The word comes from Latin meaning "to care."

OVULATION The act of expulsion of an egg (*ovum;* plural is *ova*) from one ovary or the other.

OXYTOCIN A substance that can make the uterus contract either during labor or after delivery.

OXYTOCIN CHALLENGE TEST (OCT) See *Fetal Stress Test* (FST).

PAPANICOLAOU (PAP) SMEAR A very important annual test for protection against cancer of the cervix. It consists of a smear taken directly from the cervix and screened by a trained cytology technician and, if abnormal, then read by a pathologist.

PARA The number of full-term pregnancies sustained by any one mother.

PERINATOLOGY Practicing a relatively new obstetrical subspecialty, perinatologists are also known as maternal-fetal specialists. They undergo extra training in order to manage high-risk pregnancies that involve serious problems of both mother and babe.

PERINEUM The anatomical area separating the vagina and the rectum.

PICA The craving for unusual foods or nonfood substances during pregnancy.

PLACENTA The fetal organ structure that invades its host (the mother) by attaching to a point in her uterine wall and performs tremendous hormonal and metabolic functions during pregnancy. Also called afterbirth.

PLACENTAL BARRIER A nebulous and probably nonexistent gate that was previously believed to keep toxic substances away from a *fetus.*

PROGESTERONE A very important pregnancy-related hormone excreted early in pregnancy by the ovary's *corpus luteum* cyst, and later by the *placenta*. It prevents expulsion of the *fetus* under ordinary circumstances.

PRONE PRESSURE SYNDROME An episode of weakness/faintness that often occurs when a pregnant woman lies flat on her back—particularly after mid-pregnancy. To stop it, she must turn to her left side, stay that way until she has fully recovered, then get up slowly with help.

PROSTAGLANDINS A group of newly discovered substances in our bodies that have profound effects on pregnancy as well as many other body systems. Various sorts of these agents are used to induce labor—or an abortion.

PRURITUS OF PREGNANCY A generalized body itching usually experienced in late pregnancy, it disappears after delivery. There may be no visible skin eruptions.

PTYALISM The production of excess saliva. Sometimes accompanies pregnancy.

REGIONALIZED CARE The United States is divided into regionalized perinatal centers, designated as:
- Class I: a delivery facility or hospital that is able to manage normal obstetrics
- Class II: units that can manage normal obstetrics as well as *cesarean sections* and certain operative complications
- Class III: highly sophisticated centers that can respond to any obstetrical challenge

At the core is a level III unit surrounded by a number of level I and II units feeding in severe obstetrical and neonatal problems.

RELAXIN An anterior pituitary hormone that causes the ligaments in the pelvic girdle (and elsewhere) to soften and give during pregnancy. This makes labor easier and walking harder.

RH FACTOR A useless protein substance present in some 85 percent of us (Rh-positive) and absent in the rest (Rh-negative). Its determination is of importance only in pregnancy and for blood transfusions.

SADDLE BLOCK A form of spinal *anesthesia* that involves only the very low abdomen and legs. It is useful for a vaginal delivery and lately, in combination with an epidural, to promote walking labor.

SHOW A bloody, mucous vaginal discharge that may occur near the onset of labor.

SICKLE CELL ANEMIA A type of anemia found only in African Americans. It may complicate pregnancy or vice versa.

SITZ BATH A tender, soothing dunking of your bottom in warm water—ideally in a tub, but sometimes, in hospitals, a little plastic bowl must suffice.

SPINAL BLOCK *Anesthesia* that is accomplished by inserting a drug directly into the spinal fluid. May achieve any level of pain relief desired.

STRIAE When the abdomen expands, its skin is stretched and produces the etched lines called striae—also called stretch marks. Often a deep bluish-purple during pregnancy, these lines fade into silvery webs afterward—but are not uniformly loved by their bearers.

SUDDEN INFANT DEATH SYNDROME (SIDS) There are many theories, but the best solution to date is to have babies sleep only on their backs. Also called crib death.

TERATOGEN A drug, substance, or energy source that can produce a physical abnormality in a *fetus*.

TETANIC UTERINE CONTRACTION A uterine *contraction* that lasts for a prolonged period of time—usually one minute or more.

TORCH SYNDROME The name given to a variety of infectious disorders that can have profound effects on a developing *fetus*.

TOXEMIA "Poisoning of pregnancy," or preeclampsia, this condition is found almost exclusively in the last third of pregnancy, producing generalized edema, high blood pressure, and albumin (protein) in the urine. The condition is now called *hypertension of pregnancy*.

TOXOPLASMOSIS Cat fever, an infection of significance only in pregnant women. Usually transmitted by cats, but also by poorly cooked pork.

TRICHOMONAS A common, very irritating, sexually transmitted vaginal infection of no serious obstetrical consequence.

ULTRASOUND Sound waves too high-pitched in frequency to be heard by us, ultrasound can penetrate human tissues without radiation risk, such as in X-rays. Machines that produce ultrasound waves are being used with increasing frequency in all medical areas today. Because of their safety, they are also being widely used in obstetrical diagnostic procedures. Using them, we are able to determine the health, location, and duration of pregnancy and its growth and development as pregnancy advances. New uses for this invaluable tool are being reported each day.

ULTRASOUND LEVEL Most ultrasound procedures are carried out with either the physician's own ultrasound equipment or as part of a regular radiology setting. This is level I technology. What is needed for more advanced analysis is a level II ultrasound clinic, which has highly sophisticated ultrasound equipment and physicians specially trained to interpret very precise, minute degrees of fetal growth, development, and well-being. Such clinics are part of a tertiary care obstetrical center and certain other specialized areas. See *regionalized care*.

UMBILICAL CORD A cord-like fetal structure connecting baby and *placenta*. Twelve to thirty-six inches in length, it contains three vessels—two arteries that pump blood into the placenta and a vein that brings blood back to the infant.

UMBILICUS Navel or belly button.

URETHRA A short tube that connects the bladder to the outside world. Empties just above the vagina.

URINALYSIS Routine urine testing for albumen, sugar, acetone, bacteria, pus, and blood. Usually performed—at least partially—at each prenatal visit.

UTERUS The womb; the reproductive organ that contains and nourishes a fetus until it is ready for expulsion—the uterus's climactic capability.

VERNIX CASEOSA A white, cheesy, waxy substance that coats the baby's skin in late pregnancy.

VIABLE The ability to survive; viability in babies, once impossible before the 28th week of pregnancy, is now being achieved between 20 and 25 weeks.

WOMB The *uterus*.

Index